The
New Technologies of
Birth and Death

The
New Technologies of
Birth and Death:
Medical, Legal and Moral Dimensions

Proceedings of the Workshop for Bishops of the United States and Canada
Sponsored by the Pope John Center Through a Grant from the Knights of
Columbus

Dallas, Texas, January 28-31, 1980

Pope John Center
St. Louis

Nihil Obstat:
    Rev. Robert F. Coerver, C.M., S.T.D.
    Censor Deputatus

Imprimatur:
    + John N. Wurm, S.T.D., Ph.D.
    Vicar General of St. Louis

September 17, 1980

The Nihil Obstat and Imprimatur are a declaration that a book or pamphlet is considered to be free from doctrinal or moral error. It is not implied that those who have granted the Nihil Obstat and Imprimatur agree with the contents, opinions or statements expressed.

Library of Congress Catalog Card Number: 80-83425
ISBN 0-935372-07-5

Distributors for the Trade:
    FRANCISCAN HERALD PRESS
    1434 West 51st St.
    Chicago, IL 60609

PREFACE

The ancient proverb, *nihil novi sub sole* (nothing new under the sun), reflects a static and stoic view of human existence. This volume describes something radically new and terribly important – the use of amazing new medical technology to influence the beginning and the ending of human lives.

Technology can neatly and cleanly eliminate tiny unborn human beings with vacuum aspirators and it can now also fertilize a new human life on a laboratory petri dish. Technology can now extend a human life almost indefinitely and end it abruptly with a painless injection.

The Judaeo-Christian understanding of human life and destiny insists that the Creator gave the human family both the capacity to develop technology and the responsibility to use it wisely.

Pope John Paul II spoke of the priority of ethics over technology in the same breath in which he spoke of the priority of persons over things and spirit over matter in his inaugural letter, *Redemptor Hominis*.

Sorting out these priorities can only become more puzzling in the years ahead as the enthusiastic advance of scientific research multiplies technological options in a geometric progression.

The Pope John XXIII Medical-Moral Research and Education Center in St. Louis seeks to assist the Church as it responds to the challenges of new technology. With the generous support of a grant from the Knights of Columbus the Pope John Center sponsored a Workshop for the bishops of the United States and Canada in late January, 1980, to consider the medical, legal, and moral dimensions of the new technologies of birth and death. Special thanks as well are tendered to Mr. Frank J. Schneider, of Pittsburgh, Pennsylvania, Member of the Board of Pope John Center, for his very great personal and financial support of the Workshop.

This volume contains the insights provided the 122 bishops in attendance at this historic and unprecedented conference by two doctors, two lawyers, and five theologians. It embraces subjects as old as abortion and contraception and as new as *in vitro* fertilization and the ovulation method of natural family planning. It reviews the new efforts to determine if human death has occurred even though vital signs are artificially maintained. And it explores the human and legal implications of withdrawing life-support technology and permitting death to occur.

Rev. Albert Moraczewski, O.P., the Vice-President for Research of the Pope John Center and a theologian who holds a science degree from the University of Chicago, wrote the introductory survey in this volume. It reflects his twenty-five years of research and analysis of the interface of technology and ethics.

The Pope John Center has prepared this book for wide circulation and serious consideration because, at least in the realm of human birth and death, the proverb *nihil novi sub sole* does not apply.

TABLE OF CONTENTS

Greetings

His Holiness,
Pope John Paul II

Dear Brothers in Our Lord Jesus Christ. It is with great hope and with great enthusiasm that I send my greetings to all of you assembled in Dallas. This important workshop sponsored by the Pope John XXIII Medical-Moral Research and Education Center and generously supported by the Knights of Columbus is a splendid initiative at the service of truth and at the service of the human person. The gathering of such a large number of Bishops from the United States and Canada manifests a consciousness of your pastoral responsibilities as authentic teachers of God's people who are called to live their Christian lives in the modern world. The theme of your deliberations, "The New Technologies of Birth and Death," touches upon complex and vexing questions of medical ethics which face the Church and all of society.

I had occasion in *Redemptor Hominis* to make the following statement: "The development of technology and development of contemporary civilization, which is marked by the ascendancy of technology, demand a proportional development of morals and ethics. For the present, this last development seems unfortunately to be always left behind."

In your giant efforts in Dallas, you are zealously echoing the sentiments of my heart, expressed last October in Washington, D.C. I do not hesitate to proclaim before you, and before the world, that all human life from the moment of conception and through all subsequent stages is sacred because life is created in the image and likeness of God. Our task is to proclaim ever more effectively this sacredness of human life. But in order to do so, we must understand the new opportunities and the new threats that are posed to the human person by ever-developing technologies.

At this important moment of history, you are called as Bishops to furnish timely leadership by examining new questions in the light of God's eternal Word and with the help offered by the Church's teachings. In this context, your reflections, aided by the physicians, theologians, and attorneys generously sharing their knowledge and experience at this Workshop, will help to contribute to that proportional development of morals and ethics which the contemporary situation so earnestly demands. Dear Brothers, this is a great and vital contribution of the servant Church of Jesus Christ to the men and women of our day.

May God bless the Pope John Center in its desire and commitment to be of service to the Magisterium of the Church and to the cause of humanity. And may the Holy Spirit direct your minds and hearts to enter more fully into the mysteries of His divine Wisdom and to be ever more inflamed with His Love. To all who are attending this meeting, and to all who have helped to make it possible, I cordially impart my Apostolic Blessing. In the name of the Father, and of the Son, and of the Holy Spirit. Amen.

Greetings

Mr. Virgil Dechant
Supreme Knight,
The Knights of Columbus

The Knights of Columbus are sincerely pleased to assist the Pope John XXIII Center in presenting this seminar on bioethical questions concerning life and death. We consider it a real privilege for two reasons. First, we felt the Knights could become involved in this program because of our historical commitment to assisting the Bishops in carrying out their apostolate, especially as it pertains to the moral issues confronting our people. As a corollary to this, because of our life insurance program it made sense to us that we should know more about these vital moral-medical problems.

The second reason stems from our belief that the Bishops of the United States and Canada should look to the Knights of Columbus as *their* organization. Many of you here have been so gracious in thanking us for our support for this program but, really, you should be thanking yourselves. It is your inspiration, your determination, your leadership, your guidance that have made and, God willing, will continue to make the Knights of Columbus what it is. Unless we can provide for you what you have the right to expect from us, we shall cease to fulfill that historical mission that was carved out over so many years by our predecessors.

So for these two reasons the Knights are very pleased to participate in this program – indeed, our mode of participation is easy. What we could not provide is the in-depth knowledge and scholarly expertise that you will benefit from over the next few days. That comes from the Pope John Center.

I hope that from this session we will learn, and others will learn, that we can work together in endeavors where some have the expertise and others the wherewithal. Together we can move forward to answer the problems that confront the Church and society today.

I am not a scientist, I am not a theologian and I am not eligible to be a Bishop, so I will depart tomorrow morning and go back to doing what I can do best. But I will leave behind Dr. John Griffin, our Supreme Physician, and I know that he will come back with a wonderful report to our Board of Directors. If indeed it is deemed wise by you, Your Excellencies, that this type of program should continue, I'm sure that the Knights will be glad to renew our partnership in this area.

I will also leave behind Elmer Von Feldt, editor of *Columbia* and well-known to you since for many years he worked for the National Catholic News Service. Elmer will be taking notes for an article in some future issue of *Columbia.*

I said a moment ago that I am not a scientist, not a theologian; but I am one thing: I'm a parent, I'm a husband and a father, father of four children. I know that it is not on the agenda for this meeting, but I would hope that, at some future seminar, time could be devoted to how best information on natural family planning could be disseminated. We have just conducted a survey through NORC on the attitudes of young Catholics. As an adjunct to that study another was prepared on the young Catholic family. Soon all of the Bishops will be provided with a synopsis of that study.

It will surprise you. There is tremendous hope out there for the young Catholic families of America and of Canada (the study embraced Canada also). But the one startling fact that bothers me is that young Catholics do not believe in the teachings laid down by *Humanae Vitae.* Here is an area where we must work together. Speaking as a husband and a parent now, I don't think our couples are aware of the breakthroughs that have been made in natural family planning. Much can be done in promoting NFP, and I can assure you, who represent the Magisterium of the Church, that the Knights stand ready and willing to help disseminate the information that is so vitally needed. When you are ready, be sure that the Knights will stand by you.

Thank you very much. I hope that the next few days will prove our good friend Bishop Bernard Law correct – that this seminar is the greatest thing that has happened in the medical-moral field in recent years.

Greetings

Mr. John E. Curley, Jr.
President, The Catholic
Health Association

I am privileged to have this opportunity to welcome you to this workshop on "The New Technologies of Birth and Death":

Not only because CHA was primarily responsible for the formation of the Pope John Center nearly nine years ago,

Not only because this workshop is a product of the creativity and initiative of the Pope John Center and of its desire to serve you,

Not even because each of you have committed almost five days to explore contemporary medical-moral dilemmas, a commitment which is singularly impressive because of the myriad other important demands for your attention.

But, principally because this workshop is a sign of the extent to which the hierarchy of the United States and Canada are joined with their respective Catholic health apostolates to care for and heal a wounded world.

The issues you will be addressing are not new, nor are they unfamiliar to you. However, you may be surprised by their intensity and by the extent to which an increasingly secular society has turned from the sacramental and teaching values of Christ and His Church.

Today, for example, it is no longer extraordinary for public policymakers to advocate that "living wills" be executed by the elderly as a Medicare cost-savings device; or, that abortion be emphasized as the less expensive alternative to birth; or, that sterilization be promoted among the poor to ease AFDC financial burdens; or, that amniocentesis is misused to detect defective, hence destructible, festuses; or, that definitions of death be liberalized to facilitate organ harvesting; or, that "quality of life" determinations reduce the number of institutionalized mental incompetents through euthanasia. Bizarre? Perhaps. However, each of these has been proposed or acted upon by a major civil authority in the United States during the past five years.

Consequently, health care is more than a ministry. It is also the forum within which our values are competing to survive. Will our values survive the competition? I believe they will. For together, whether as pastors or as ministers, we bring to health care and to the people we care for, a value tradition rooted in the gospels and premised upon the sanctity of each human life and the dignity of each human person. Through our love, compassion, and service, we bring Christ! And, Christ is ultimately undeniable.

I trust in the presence of Christ at this workshop. And, on behalf of The Catholic Health Association of the United States, I wish you the kind of workshop experience that I know you will have.

Introduction

Dominion, Bioethics and Pluralism

Reverend Albert S. Moraczewski, O.P., Ph.D.

Introduction

With majestic simplicity the author of Genesis proclaims:

> God created man in his image;
> in the divine image he created him;
> male and female he created them.
> God blessed them, saying: "Be fertile
> and multiply; fill the earth and subdue
> it. Have dominion over the fish of the
> sea, the birds of the air, and all living
> things that move on the earth" (Gen. 1:27-28).

What awesome beauty and wisdom are contained in those few words! Deep in his mysterious counsels, God has chosen to create us in his image and to share dominion over the world he has created. So great a dignity concomitantly places on us a great responsibility to exercise that dominion wisely.

The Human Race and Technological Progress

Gradual Control Over Nature: Gradually, over untold millennia, the human race has understood with increasing depth of knowledge the world on which it has been placed. Bit by bit, we have struggled to gain mastery over the forces of nature: fire for warmth and cooking; clothes for protection against the cold and for decorative purposes; weapons to hunt for food and to protect against enemies; tools to fashion a variety of items including implements for cultivation and for the construction of shelters. We have tamed animals to serve our needs; we have found substances in plants and animals to cure diseases, to relieve pain, to produce sleep or euphoria – all to help overcome the rigors and tedium of life.

Amazing Technological Feats of Today: At an increasing rate our ability to control nature and its forces has led to the amazing feats which characterize the present age: radio, satellite communication; television, automobiles, jet planes; space travel to the moon and beyond; clothes, buildings, utensils, toys and books, all in infinite variety of colors and shapes; computers which execute millions of mathematical operations a second, computers so small that a paper clip is large by comparison; computers which control business operations, government decisions, traffic, and work out theoretical problems in physics, chemistry, biochemistry; computers which simulate human intelligence. With optical and radio telescopes, we have peered into the vast distances of space and in doing so have also seen the remote past history of the universe, even perhaps its birth (though not its creative conception) in a gigantic pregnant explosion. Optical microscopes supplemented by electron microscopes have given us a view of the microcosm that constitutes a single cell – the intricate structure, the harmonious complexity of biochemical reactions interacting at lightning speed yet each delicately and precisely achieving its respective end. What beauty therein lies! How God's wisdom shines forth in his creation at all levels! The mighty cyclotrons and synchrotons have opened to us the door of the atom's structure only to reveal that there exist substructures within the atomic particles.

From the subatomic spheres to the outermost reaches of space, humans have probed and peered, both to understand and to control. In the relentless search for knowledge and mastery human beings have not spared themselves. The human body and mind has been poked, cut, removed, replaced, and made whole. Numerous illnesses – but not all – have been conquered. Human life at both ends of the spectrum has been studied: how does it begin? How does it end? What can we do to control life's beginning? Not satisfied with understanding the processes of generation and gestation, we humans are now seeking to specify the bodily and mental characteristics of the human persons who will be generated. Fearful of death, we search to slow down the inevitable aging and dying. We want to control the manner of our death; we want to be able to lay down our life and take it up again – on our terms!

The Church and Technological Progress

The Church Not Opposed to Technology: The official teaching of the Church, it should be emphasized, is clearly not opposed to the proper use of technology. Pope John XXIII had declared in his encyclicals *Mater et Magistra* and *Pacem in Terris:*

> For it is indeed clear that the Church always taught and continues to teach that advances in science and technology and the prosperity resulting therefrom, are truly to be counted as good things and regarded as signs of the progress of civilization. But the Church likewise teaches that goods of this kind are to be judged properly in accordance with their natures: they are always to be considered as instruments for man's use, the better to achieve his highest end: that he can then the more easily improve himself, and in both the natural and supernatural orders *(Mater et Magistra, #246)*. But the progress of science and the inventions of technology show above all the infinite greatness of God, Who created the universe and man himself *(Pacem in Terris, #3)*.

The Second Vatican Council in *Gaudium et Spes* reveals a positive attitude toward science:

> Man has always striven to develop his life through his mind and his work; today his efforts have achieved a measure of success, for he has extended and continues to extend his mastery over nearly all spheres of nature thanks to science and technology *(Gaudium et Spes, #33)*. Far from considering the conquests of man's genius and courage as opposed to God's power as if he set himself up as a rival to the creator, Christians ought to be convinced that the achievements of the human race are a sign of God's greatness and the fulfillment of his mysterious design *(Gaudium et Spes, #34)*.

Most recently, the writings and addresses of Pope John Paul have indicated continued interest in, and support of, science. In his address to the Pontifical Academy of Science on November 10, 1979, Pope

John Paul reiterated his respect for science and at the same time made an important distinction between pure and applied science:

> The search for truth is the task of basic science. The researcher who moves on this first versant of science, feels all the fascination of St. Augustine's words: "Intellectum valde ama" (Epist. 120, 3, 13; PL 33, 459), "he loves intelligence" and the function that is characteristic of it, to know truth. Pure science is good, which every people must be able to cultivate in full freedom from all forms of international slavery or intellectual colonialism.
>
> Basic research must be free with regard to the political and economic authorities, which must cooperate in its development, without hampering it in its creativity or harnessing it to serve their own purposes. Like any other truth, scientific truth is, in fact, answerable only to itself and to the supreme Truth, God, the creator of man and of all things *(L'Osservatore Romano,* November 26, 1979, p. 9, No. 2).
>
> On its second versant, science turns to practical applications, which find their full development in the various technologies. In the phase of its concrete achievements, science is necessary to mankind to satisfy the rightful requirements of life, and to overcome the different ills that threaten it. There is no doubt that applied science has rendered and will continue to render immense services to man, provided it is inspired by love, regulated by wisdom, and accompanied by the courage that defends it against the undue interference of all tyrannical powers. Applied science must be united with conscience, so that, in the trinomial, science-technology-conscience, it is the cause of man's real good that is served *(L'Osservatore Romano,* November 26, 1979, p. 9, No. 3).

Moral Concerns Regarding Technology

Yet not all is well with the way we have responded to God's command to subdue the earth. There are signs, ecological and human, that something is wrong. The question needs to be asked again: what are the limits of our dominion? When are we reaching for the forbidden fruit? The technological mastery which is now in our hands requires a proportionate *moral* control. As great as are the achievements of modern science and technology, they are, as Pope John Paul II pointed out in his encyclical, *Redemptor Hominis* (#16), subject to the judgment of ethical principles. These technological achievements must be truly in service of human persons; they must contribute to the establishment and maintenance of peace and justice on earth, and thus ultimately serve the Kingdom of God.

The urgency of the challenge to moral dominion over technology requires that the task not be delayed any further. But the vastness and complexity of the problem compels us to limit the scope of our inquiry to some aspects of biomedical technology. Accordingly, this workshop will focus on two areas:

1. The beginning of individual human life
2. The end of individual human existence on earth.

This overview will consider the value issues in biomedical technology within these two areas and will outline the pluralism of moral methodologies used within the Church to respond to these value issues.

I. Value Issues in Biomedical Technology

Issues and Technologies Surrounding Conception and Birth

Reproductive Technologies: Human control over conception, gestation and birth has increased steadily in the past decades. The crudest sort of control is simply to terminate the existence of a human being, to abort a living child. A less destructive form of control is to prevent the conception of a human being by any one of a variety of chemicals and devices. Greater technological skill is reflected in the use of artificial insemination, *in vitro* fertilization, and embryo transplants to assist in sexual reproduction. A refinement would be the employment of genetic engineering techniques to produce a child with specific genetic traits or one free from selected genetic diseases. Perhaps the ultimate in technological accomplishments would be the nonsexual reproduction of human beings by means of cloning. This last term refers to a technique which, in theory at least, would permit individuals to reproduce genetically identical copies of themselves, a younger carbon copy, so to speak.

Abortion Technologies: Of the above technological applications clearly the one which in our time presents the gravest and most urgent moral problem is, of course, abortion. While abortion and infanticide have been practiced for millennia in various cultures and societies, it is our current civilization which has enlisted the resources of modern technology to insure a more efficient destruction of the unborn child while at the same time making the procedure safer for the woman, and sad to say, more lucrative for participating physicians and certain

7

industries. When we consider that there were over one million abortions performed in the United States in 1978, the magnitude of such slaughter appalls us.

Articles in obstetrical journals often describe the various techniques of abortion currently available as well as discussing which procedures are more efficacious and safe at different stages of pregnancy. The latest technique involves the injection of a substance naturally present in human tissues called prostaglandin (because it was first identified in the seminal fluid and also found in extracts of prostate glands). Certain forms of this substance (PGF2D) have the ability to bring about a contraction of the uterus and are used to induce labor. When the child is not able to survive outside its mother's womb induction of labor is an abortion. The goal of abortion research is to produce a substance which can be self-administered at home and which will effectively and safely abort a child within the first six weeks after a missed menstrual period.

The older procedures of aborting such as those done by removing the pregnant uterus, by doing a Caesarian section and emptying the uterus, by sucking out the contents of the pregnant uterus with a vacuum apparatus, and by destroying the child in the uterus by injecting a 20% saline solution into the uterus, were all considered less than desirable. Consequently, the prostaglandin technique was welcomed. However, an unwelcome consequence in the use of prostaglandin is that on occasion a live child is delivered.

Side by side with the development of newer procedures for abortion is the change in attitude on the part of many obstetricians, especially since January 22, 1973. Abortion then became part of physician's armamentarium. Reasons for abortion were not restricted to saving a mother's life but were extended to include any threat to her health. Such abortions were verbally ennobled with the term *"therapeutic"* abortions. Under the aegis of an accepted medical procedure, abortions could be performed for almost any reason and, it would seem, even merely on demand from a pregnant woman. As to the physician, he or she could interpret "therapeutic need" to include any situation which held out the possibility of injuring— even slightly— the physical or mental or emotional social health of the patient. Consequently, if abortion was seen as a means of restoring or preserving the health of the woman, it could then be invoked as a therapeutic abortion.

Contraception Technologies: Distinct, but not entirely unrelated, are the issues surrounding contraception. In the contemporary western culture even weightier than abortion are the financial implications for certain pharmaceutical manufacturers of contraceptive drugs and devices such as the IUD (Intra Uterine Device). The annual market value runs in the millions of dollars. While various forms of earlier contraceptive devices such as the condom, diaphragm, jelly, foams and the like are still being employed, until very recent times the most popular were the different combinations of estrogens and progesterones – natural and synthetic – used to control ovulation. When the undesirable side effects of these substances were discovered and made known to the general public, there was understandably a reaction on the part of women against their use. One result of this situation, together with the impact of the woman's liberation movement, was to urge the development of *male* contraceptives. After extensive animal studies which showed that these substances, when effective, inhibit the formation of viable spermatazoa, clinical testing on volunteer male human subjects was undertaken. As yet it is too early to state whether and to what degree success may have been attained.

Another reaction to the news about the possible deleterious impact on the women's health or life of the "Pill" was a return – by some – to practices of earlier times. One of these, the cervical cap, recently has been improved by work done by a dentist at the University of Chicago. Using the insights and skills associated with the making of caps and crowns for teeth, he custom-makes a cervical cap for each patient by making an impression of the woman's cervix with dental impression material from which cast the contraceptive device is fashioned. This procedure insures that the cap fits snugly over the cervix and that it functions as an effective barrier to the transport of sperm.

One of the ideals sought for in the area of contraceptives is to find one which can also act *after* intercourse. Some have been dubbed the "morning-after pill." The copper-coated IUDs are thought to act effectively for five days after intercourse. The problem with these late-acting devices and chemicals is that in all likelihood they function as abortifacients. Thus, it has been well said that the ultimate in contraceptives is abortion; it is the back-up procedure when the "main line" contraceptives fail to deliver. A means of controlling conception

9

which does not have most of the adverse reactions associated with the "Pill" and with IUDs, is that included in the term Natural Family Planning (NFP). The technology does not require the use of any drugs or devices. NFP is based primarily on certain physiological signs associated with ovulation and on the utilization of certain naturally inherent cycles of the body.

Pro-conception Technologies: Apart from contraceptive procedures and abortion, artificial insemination, the first technological intervention in the conception process, was introduced at the beginning of the 19th century. Artificial insemination was successfully done on animals from the late 1700's. After an early initial attempt on human beings, the practice did not begin in earnest until the middle of the 19th century. According to one report, in the United States alone some 10,000 persons a year are born who have been conceived with the use of *donor* sperm. Our century has added the technique of freezing the human sperm. Within the past few years sperm banks have been established in the United States and throughout the world: twelve in the U.S., fifteen in France, and about ten in other countries. At least 3,000 persons world-wide have already been conceived with the use of *frozen* sperm, generally donor sperm. Because of genetic concerns, some physicians expressed strong reservations about the use of frozen donor sperm when it was reported that at least one individual male donor has sired fifty children through the use of frozen sperm. In addition, the storing in the deep freeze of frozen human eggs and frozen human embryos for thawing at a convenient time are other possibilities being discussed.

What the science-fiction writers had written years ago became a reality when Louise Brown was born on July 24, 1978 after having been conceived in a small laboratory dish – a Petri plate. The media immediately labeled her a "test-tube baby," an appellation both incorrect and pejorative. She spent about 2½ days in a glass-enclosed environment before being introduced into the womb of her mother where she spent the next 8½ months. The "success" of this conception and birth should not obscure the fact that years of research and experimentation by Drs. Patrick Steptoe and Robert Edwards had preceded the birth of Louise Brown nor should it be overlooked that possibly more than one hundred human lives were destroyed. These lives had been tiny human embryos (human beings) which had been conceived in an artificial environment and either discarded for one reason or another, or had been unable to achieve or to maintain implantation and so rejected by the mother's body.

The process which brought about the conception of Louise Brown is sometimes termed *"in vitro* fertilization." This expression in itself refers only to the manner in which the egg and sperm are brought together. Placing the resulting embryo into a woman's uterus is termed "embryo transplant." However, as a kind of shorthand, *"in vitro* fertilization" sometimes denotes the entire process from obtaining the human egg and sperm, bringing them together and, after a suitable time for development, placing the resulting embryo in the uterus of a woman. For this process the sperm may be donated by the husband of the woman or by another, and the woman who receives the embryo may or may not be the same person who produced the egg.

Because the process is divisible, the human embryo may be allowed to come to term and birth. Alternatively, the human embryo may be allowed to grow in an artificial environment and be used as a subject for research. Many see this as an opportunity to study the physiological, biochemical and anatomical changes that occur in the earliest stages of embryological development. Such studies could provide valuable insights into the nature of normal and abnormal human fetal development. In the latter case, a deeper and more accurate understanding of the relative contributions of genetic defects and environmental toxins to birth defects could be obtained. Pharmacological studies on the developing human embryo could discover adverse effects of drugs on the human fetus before they are prescribed for pregnant women. Eventually the technological means to carry a human fetus the entire nine months to term in a fully artificial environment will be discovered. When that process becomes a reality, we will have reached the situation which Aldous Huxley described exactly fifty years ago in his *Brave New World:* children mass-produced in a laboratory.

Human-animal Hybrids: While human-animal hybrids clearly are not on the horizon, research has already been done involving the joining or fusing of human and animal cells. Man and mouse cells have been fused in tissue cultures but because of the great differences in genetic constitution such cells are not capable of perduring for any length of time nor of reproducing themselves beyond one or two cell-divisions.

Attempts at cross-fertilizing animal egg cells with human sperm have found that there are normally at least two cellular barriers which prevent a foreign sperm from entering the egg and fusing with its nucleus. Cross-breeding among animals does not occur in their natural habitats primarily because of behavioral and territorial barriers. Only in the artificial conditions of the laboratory do foreign eggs and sperm get the opportunity to meet. Nothing in the scientific literature suggests that any serious attempts have been made to bring about human/animal fertilization with the intent of producing an offspring.

Non-sexual Reproduction: Finally, mention should be made – even if only for completion – of another reproductive technique, cloning. This technique may be briefly described as a form of non-sexual reproduction. One form requires that an unfertilized egg cell have its nucleus removed and replaced by the nucleus from any body cell. Given the proper conditions, the resulting egg cell, having the full complement of genetic information, is theoretically capable of dividing and developing into a genetically identical copy of the person from whom the replacement nucleus has been obtained.

Although this technique apparently was successfully carried out some fifteen years ago with frogs, no convincing evidence has been published regarding the cloning of any higher form of life. Claims of cloning mice have not been fully accepted. Consequently, any claims, especially by novelists, that human cloning is in the near future should be viewed with considerable skepticism.

Genetic Diagnostic Techniques: Other techniques related to medical problems arising during pregnancy such as those relating to genetics are important but will not be the explicit focus of this workshop. Amniocentesis used to obtain fluid from the amniotic sac of a pregnant woman in order to study the condition of the fetus is one of the principal techniques in this area. Fetoscopy is a technique which permits one to see inside the pregnant woman and directly observe the fetus. Sonography uses high-frequency sound waves to determine the size, parts, location and orientation of the fetus in the mother's womb without invading the body of the mother. It is used often in conjunction with the other two techniques mentioned above in order to lessen the danger of harming the fetus when the instruments are introduced into the amniotic sac.

Moral Issues Associated with Conception and Birth Technologies

Notwithstanding some of the positive contributions which many of these reproductive technologies may be able to make, there are grave moral issues surrounding their usage which cannot be lightly dismissed. At the same time their novelty should not of itself be the cause of an immediate and absolute prohibition. The values which each particular technological application threatens (or protects) need to be identified.

Since many of the moral issues mentioned here will be treated much more fully in the subsequent presentations of this workshop, the primary concern in this essay will be to suggest some of the issues and values at risk.

Clearly, the current major moral issue in the area of reproductive technologies is abortion. The value at stake is human life. While other lesser rights (values) such as the right to health of the mother, her right to privacy, etc., may be in conflict, the law of the land clearly permits these latter rights to supervene over the unborn child's right to life. A further complication arises when one considers a Catholic physician or nurse, a Catholic health facility, or a bishop when each respectively is confronted with the legality of "therapeutic" abortion. How are the rights of the respective consciences of parties in conflict to be honored?

Some of the contraceptive techniques bring about their desired effect by preventing successful implantation: these are, in effect, abortifacients. The primary effect apparently of the IUDs is to prevent implantation of the fertilized egg. Substances such as the "Pill" have several effects, one of which is to suppress ovulation; another renders the lining of the uterus hostile to implantation.

In connection with "pro-conception" technologies the equivalency of abortion appears. *In vitro* fertilization and embryo transplant both entail the exposure of the living human embryo to life-threatening conditions. Indeed, during the development of this technology numerous human embryos have been deliberately destroyed or have been placed in an environment which made their survival highly problematical or impossible.

Another set of moral concerns centers around the marital act. Under what conditions, if any, may we intervene in the marital act? Such intervention may be either to *prevent* conception or to *assist* it. In the former, prevention of conception may be either permanent, such as is brought about by surgical sterilization, or it may be temporary as with the chemical and mechanical contraceptives. If technology is to assist conception then what are the conditions, if any, and in what manner may we intervene? These concerns apply to such technologies as artificial insemination, both by husband's sperm (AIH) and by donor sperm (AID), to *in vitro* fertilization, and to embryo transplant.

A long-range moral issue in the area of reproduction has to do with the limits of our dominion in this area. May we attempt to reproduce by non-sexual means? As previously described, cloning is the term applied to non-sexual reproduction. Are there situations where resort to this type of reproduction would be morally permissible? Granted that the realization of such technology is probably more distant in the future than its enthusiasts had predicted, should efforts even be initiated to accomplish such a reproductive technology?

Finally, a set of moral concerns are to be found in the area of human fetal experimentation. In particular, it is a question of doing research on very young human embryos (less than 14 days old) which, under certain conditions, the Department of Health, Education and Welfare's Ethics Advisory Board had approved. May the parents, or the courts, ever give approval for non-therapeutic research on living human embryos? These and other moral questions will be treated in more detail in subsequent essays in this volume.

Issues and Technologies Surrounding Death and Dying

Death as the Cessation of Respiration and Heart Beat: In some ways the varieties of technologies and moral issues surrounding death are less complex than those associated with conception and death. Heretofore people died rather simply. Once the natural forces of the human body were no longer able to function in an integrative manner due to trauma, disease or old age, the person simply died. There was not much fellow human beings could do to stop the dying process or to delay it significantly. Death generally was recognized by, and identified as, the cessation of respiration and heartbeat. No sophisticated instrumentation was available, or needed to make the determination of death.

Blood Transfusions: Now in 1980, medicine has a vast array of techniques, instruments, and medication to stave off death. Blood and plasma transfusion can be administered when the person has lost a significant amount of blood. Very recently, a synthetic, non-blood substitute has been developed – but not yet medically approved – for

14

life-saving purposes when the patient cannot tolerate another person's blood for physiological or religious reasons.

Antibiotics: A major source of death in the past has been infections which have overwhelmed the body's natural defenses. Roughly since World War II when effective antibiotics were developed, deaths resulting from infections have been drastically reduced.

Improved Surgical and Nursing Procedures: Surgical procedures have greatly improved, especially since the introduction of general anesthetics in the middle of last century which permitted longer and more complex operations. One result has been a decrease in the incidence of death resulting from accidents and other causes. These surgical procedures have been supplemented by skilled medical and nursing care which not only made recovery from surgery more assured but also in many cases supported or revived the will to live on the part of the patient.

Organ Transplantation: Such techniques as organ transplantation, especially kidney transplantation, have added to the life span of a number of persons. More dramatic, of course, have been the heart transplantations which were inaugurated in the middle 1960's. For a variety of reasons heart transplantation is still not widely employed. In a few medical centers the procedure is carried out with varying degrees of success. Dr. Shumway and others at Stanford University, for example, continue to perform these operations and have performed 181 heart transplantations since 1968. Having learned from earlier experiences of others as well as his own, Shumway has formulated rigid criteria for the selection of heart recipients and donors so as to maximize the chances of a successful transplant. Other organ transplantations, such as liver and pancreas, have been tried but with rather poor success. Bone marrow transplantations have been somewhat more successful. In all these areas additional basic and clinical research and experience are required.

Prostheses: Closely related to organ transplantations is the use of artificial limbs and organs (known as prostheses). In terms of life-saving devices some progress has been made with heart, kidney and lung substitutes. Of the three organs mentioned, the heart seems to be the easiest to construct since it is primarily a "pump," although more problems have arisen than apparently had been anticipated. As a consequence no one – as far as I know – is walking around with an artificial heart buried in his or her chest. More difficult to duplicate are the kidneys, because, in part, the kidney performs complex chemical reactions during the process of removing from the blood the waste products of metabolic activity. More successful has been an *external* kidney, commonly known as the "kidney machine" or chronic hemodialysis or kidney dialysis. Persons with temporary or permanent kidney failure, who previously would have died quickly, are now able to live longer. The demand both for these machines to which a patient needs to be hooked up for several hours three or four times a week and for kidneys for transplantation purposes exceeds the supply, especially with regard to the natural kidney. These problems are examples of the larger issues of the allocation of scarce resources.

Artificial Life Support Systems: In the public eye, the most telling sign of life prolongation perhaps is the artificial life-support system. One part of the system is the mechanical respirator which takes over the task of breathing when the individual cannot breathe spontaneously. Injections of stimulant drugs may also be used to maintain the heart beat. Oxygen may be supplied to insure adequate oxygen supply to the tissues even though mechanical respiratory support is being given.

Techniques for Pain Relief: In addition to the above armamentarium which a physician has available to save the patient's life, modern medical technology has developed a variety of drugs as well as surgical and electronic techniques to reduce the pain of cancer and other diseases, and of traumas due to accidents. Reduction of pain in some instances will extend the individual's life as well as making human communication more possible.

Moral Issues Associated with Death and Dying Technologies

Three sets of issues are associated with the use of these technologies:
1. Moral issues surrounding the determination of death
2. Moral issues surrounding the decision whether to use or not use life saving procedures
3. Moral issues surrounding the deliberate termination of life, i.e., euthanasia.

Each of these will be briefly considered at this point.

Determination of Death: A relatively new dimension in the area of death and dying has to do with the criteria for death. In the majority of instances, cessation of spontaneous respiration and heart beat are

16

perfectly adequate signs of death. However, when the patient is receiving artificial life support the very equipment and procedures makes the application of those relatively simple criteria very difficult or impossible.

A further complication in the determination of death has been the introduction of organ transplant technology which requires that in the interest in having the organs in the most useful condition, it is mandatory that these be removed as quickly after death as possible. All other things being equal, a kidney or heart from a living patient is preferable to one from a cadaver. At the same time the heart and both kidneys may not be removed from a living person. Consequently, the donor must have died and been declared dead before these organs may be removed. The requirement for "freshest" organs places a pressure on the attending physician to make the determination of death as quickly and accurately as possible.

For the above and other reasons, substitute criteria for death have been sought. Most popular have been the so-called "brain death" criteria. A number of specific sets of criteria (e.g., the Harvard criteria) for determining whether the brain is dead have been developed but differ in detail. All criteria, however, proceed on the assumption that death of the brain is equivalent to death of the person: if the brain is dead, John Doe is dead. Some have contested this concept as not being certain. Others have pointed out the ambiguity in the expression "brain death." What does it mean to say the brain is dead? What part of the brain? All of it? For how long must it be dead? What are suitable medical criteria for such a determination? These and other questions, some of which are medical and others philosophical, have been raised and must be considered as part of the total area of concern about death and dying.

To Use or Not to Use Life-Saving Procedures: Some persons have a fear – not entirely without foundation – that unreasonable efforts will be made to keep them alive when it is morally permissible not to use certain means to continue life needlessly. Physicians with some concern about malpractice suits are hesitant in not using all technological resources at hand to maintain life. Soaring medical and hospitalization costs have added still another dimension to the moral problem.

The opposite situation is also a concern: the patient or family wishes the life-saving efforts continued when the physician states that medically there is little or no hope for survival or regaining consciousness. Or, in opposition to the desires of the family, the physician responds to the expressed earlier wish of the patient to discontinue efforts at life support when there is no reasonable hope of benefit. What moral principles are useful to resolve these problems? In what manner is the traditional principle of double effect to be understood and applied in these situations? In final analysis, *who* makes the decision to use or not use life-saving procedures?

Euthanasia: While etymologically the word "euthanasia" means simply a good death, in actual usage the term is equivalent to "mercy killing." The latter sense will be used in these presentations. Mercy killing refers to the deliberate action by which a person's life is brought to an end; in effect, the person is either killed or commits suicide. Injecting a massive dose of morphine or taking knowingly a large overdose of a sleep-producing drug like a barbiturate are examples. Not using available life-sustaining means when one has the obligation to do so is a form of euthanasia.

What moral principles are applicable here? Are there any situations where a person might freely and with moral rectitude submit to euthanasia? Persons watching someone they love dying with intolerable pain have concluded that it is an act of love and therefore morally acceptable to hasten death in such extreme situations. Can such a conclusion ever be morally justified?

The Use of Moral Principles

In brief fashion we have surveyed the technologies involved with the beginning and end of life. These technological innovations are merely an extension of what the human race has been doing for millennia, namely, gaining control over the forces of nature to use them for human needs and purposes. However, these inventions and discoveries must be regulated by moral principles to insure that they serve truly the well-being of human beings. Because of the complexity of the issues and weakness of the human spirit living in a world which has known sin, moral evaluations of these issues made by theologians and ethicists have differed. In particular, in American Catholic moral theology there are currently two principal methods for making a moral evaluation of such problems. One, the traditional method, seems reflected in and presupposed by Magisterial teachings. This method holds that there are moral principles applicable to the conjugal act and to innocent human life which are exceptionless. The other methodology holds that there are no such principles because the specific circumstances surrounding the act are significant moral determinants in the weighing of values and disvalues. The act considered in itself cannot be judged to be morally good or evil; the act in the abstract can only have a premoral or ontic evil.

The morality of the various technologies described in the preceding sections in many cases will be judged differently depending on which moral methodology is used. Consequently, it is necessary at this point to give some consideration to the problem of pluralism of moral methodologies in the Church.

II. Pluralism of Moral Methodologies

While not denying the reality of the divisions in moral theology within the Church, many persons deplore this state of affairs. The concern is not merely that theologians disagree with one another; rather it is that some theologians are openly critical of the teaching of the Magisterium on a number of moral issues where previously there had been unanimity. The issue of pluralism cannot be ignored nor simply dismissed out of hand. What is needed first is an understanding of what seems to some to be the major elements.

Magisterial Teaching: For our present needs there are two teachings which are most relevant: (1) that regarding the inviolability of human life, and (2) that concerning the conjugal act. In connection with the sacredness of human life, the words of John Paul II delivered at the Washington Mall during his 1979 visit to the United States summarize briefly what has been the constant teaching of the Church.

> I do not hesitate to proclaim before you and before the world that all human life – from the moment of conception and through all subsequent stages – is sacred, because human life is created in the image and likeness of God . . . And so, we will stand up every time that human life is threatened.
>
> – when the sacredness of life before birth is attacked we will stand up and proclaim that no one ever has the authority to destroy unborn life (*Origins* 9, 18:279-80).

According to this teaching, human life, innocent of any serious crime, may never directly and deliberately be taken. No combination of good intentions and circumstances can convert the evil action of unjust killing into a morally good act.

The teaching of the Magisterium concerning the conjugal act has been stated and restated clearly by recent pontiffs. Pius XI stated: "Any use whatsoever of matrimony exercised in such a way that the act is deliberately frustrated in its natural power to generate life is an offense against the law of God and of nature, and those who indulge in such are branded with the guilt of grave sin" *(Casti Connubii)*.

This teaching was continued and reiterated vigorously by Pope Pius XII as for example:

> But the Church has likewise rejected the opposite attitude which would pretend to separate, in generation, the biological activity in the personal relation of the married couple. . . . It is in the unity of this human act that we should consider the biological conditions of generation. Never is it permitted to separate these various aspects to the positive exclusion either of the procreative intention or of the conjugal relationship (*Linacre Quarterly* 46, 4:311).

The Second Vatican Council also took up this topic even if its words were somewhat attenuated by the realization that Paul VI had directed that a full discussion of the issue was to be reserved to him. Nonetheless, the teaching is clear:

> When it is a question of harmonizing married love with the responsible transmission of life, it is not enough to take only the good intention and the evaluation of motives into account; the objective criteria must be used, criteria drawn from the nature of the human person and human action, . . . In questions of birth regulation the sons of the Church, faithful to these principles, are forbidden to use methods disapproved of by the teaching authority of the Church in its interpretation of the divine law (*Gaudium et Spes, #51*).

In response to various attacks on the Church's teaching on conjugal morality, Paul VI stated in his encyclical *Humanae Vitae,* and repeated in a number of subsequent addresses, the Church's teaching ". . . each and every marriage act (*quilibet matrimonii usus*) must remain open to the transmission of life" (#11).

From these few quotations it is apparent that the Magisterium will not countenance any exemptions to both moral principles: the inviolability of innocent human life, and the non-divisibility of procreative and unitive functions in the marital act. The exceptionless nature of these principles is what the dissenters question. The following section seeks to summarize their position on these issues.

Dissent from the Magisterial Teaching: Fundamentally, the dissent centers around the nature of the human act from a moral point of view. Traditionally, the morality of a human act was considered to involve three components: the moral object (i.e., the act itself considered in the abstract), the intention, and the circumstances. The overall morality of a concrete human act required that each component be considered *separately;* each component had to be morally good or at least neutral. Good intentions or allegedly extenuating circumstances could not override an evil moral object; if that were evil then the total, concrete human act would be judged as morally evil.

New Moral Methodology: The proponents of the new methodology hold that human act must be determined by these three components taken *simultaneously.* From this perspective, no act considered in the abstract can be intrinsically evil. This position denies that there are any absolute moral norms; every moral rule may have some exception given the right combination of moral object, circumstances and intention. Accordingly the morality of any concrete human action is determined by a balancing or weighing of the various values and disvalues associated with that particular act. If the values outweigh the disvalues, the act is morally good; if disvalues have the greater weight, then the action is judged to be morally evil.

Applying this new moral methodology to the moral issues at hand, one can readily see that the moral evaluation might sometimes differ from that of the Magisterium. By denying the universally binding applicability of the two moral principles mentioned above and taught by the Magisterium, those holding the new methodology are led to conclude, in principle at least, that there can be a combination of intentions and circumstances which would, in some cases, morally permit abortion, sterilization, contraception, *in vitro* fertilization, embryo transplants, and cloning.

Nature of the Dissent: Existence of dissent reflects a certain dissatisfaction with the traditional moral methodology. That dissatisfaction may have been a reaction to the manner in which natural law arguments were employed. However, there were other reasons too, stemming from an increasing awareness of the complexity of current moral problems in a highly technological society.

The complexity of current moral problems has its roots partly in the realization that human moral decisions are influenced by many factors. Insights provided by Freud, Adler, Jung and others have shown how precarious is human freedom, how many psychosocial factors shape human decisions. Traditional moral theology recognized the enemies of freedom – strong emotions, ignorance, for example – but today there is a realization that these enemies are more numerous, hidden, and pervasive than previously appreciated.

Other roots of the moral complexity are to be found in the complexity of modern life, and in the impact of personal decisions on societal concerns. Altogether, it is concluded by some that the inherent complexity of moral questions makes it impossible to exclude all possibility of error. Consequently, the Magisterium, from this viewpoint, is simply not able to assert such official teaching to be absolutely true.

One motivating factor, they claim, which has urged theologians to seek different solutions from those taught by the Magisterium has been a more intense and personal awareness of pastoral needs. The experience of several recent wars has underlined for many the primacy of persons over institutions. Traditionally, even if unspoken, there was a tendency to subordinate the individual to the institution. To protect, for example, the institution of marriage it was considered better for some individuals to suffer than to permit divorce with remarriage in cases where grounds for annulment could not be adequately established.

The Magisterium and theologians who support it have reacted strongly to the dissenters by insisting on the right of the Magisterium to make definitive interpretations of the Gospel and of the natural law. Clearly, there is no question that the official teachers of faith and morals can and do learn from the theologians and other persons. Nonetheless, the question remains: who is to decide which teaching is in accord or not in accord with the faith the Church has received? From its inception the Church has clearly and steadfastly held that the touchstone of faith is the faith and morals held by the Pope and the bishops united to him. Ultimately, it would seem that, while theologians can suggest, urge, criticize, analyze, and propose, at some point the Magisterium must state unambiguously whether a teaching is or is not in accord with the received faith.

The Magisterium can do so because it has received this mandate from the Lord and exercises it under the guidance of the Holy Spirit:

But the task of giving an authentic interpretation of the Word of

God, whether in its written form or in the form of tradition, has been entrusted to the living teaching office of the Church alone. Its authority in this matter is exercised in the name of Jesus Christ (*Dei Verbum,* #10).

Not only has the Magisterium competency to interpret the Word of God, but also the natural moral law:

No believer will wish to deny that the teaching authority of the Church is competent to interpret even the natural moral law. It is, in fact, indisputable, as our predecessors have many times declared, that Jesus Christ, when communicating to Peter and to the Apostles His divine authority and sending them to teach all nations his Commandments, constituted them as guardians and authentic interpreters of all the moral law, not only, that is, of the law of the Gospel, but also of the natural law, which is also an expression of the will of God, the faithful fulfillment of which is equally necesary for salvation (*Humanae Vitae,* #4).

Finally in matters of faith and morals the faithful are to give a sincere assent to the teaching authority of the Church:

This loyal submission of the will and intellect must be given, in a special way, to the authentic teaching authority of the Roman Pontiff, even when he does not speak *ex cathedra* . . . (*Lumen Gentium,* #25).

While theological conflicts can be sharp and intense, all parties to this controversy are presumed to be persons of good will – unless there is clear evidence to the contrary. They are Christians attempting to deal with complex moral issues fraught with human pain. Those who support Magisterial teaching as well as those who oppose it on some points are seeking earnestly to be faithful to the message of Jesus Christ. All parties are convinced that their particular moral methodology better preserves and promotes Gospel values. So then, how is the truth to be ascertained? When individuals and groups are making contradictory statements, both cannot be correct. What can be done to alleviate the situation? Clearly the Christian people are puzzled by conflicting claims, and moral life is troubled by the unsettled conditions. Reconciliation must be sought; the first step in that process is for all parties to desire and seek a clear understanding of what the other is saying. Equally or more important is to determine what may be the underlying assumptions which govern the respective methodologies. Out of this process should be born a deeper understanding of the issues and a firmer grasp of the relevant moral principles.

Conclusion

The essays presented in this volume should be viewed against the background just presented. The essays themselves do not resolve the underlying issues of theological methodology. What they do accomplish is to provide a discussion of specific bioethical issues in the context of that contemporary discussion.

The workshop for which these essays were prepared was designed to provide a suitable process for analyzing the moral problems presented by the new technologies surrounding birth and death in the light of the relevant papal teachings. Included also was the objective of providing current and critically evaluated medical and legal information applicable to these topics. Within the moral analysis, primacy was to be given to the viewpoint which was most in accord with what the Magisterium has promulgated. Nonetheless, other perspectives would not be excluded from consideration. No theologian would be attacked or denigrated. What was sought was a workable response to problems complex in their ethical structure and very painful in their human dimension.

This introductory chapter has previewed the value issues raised by the use of new technology in connection with human birth and death and outlined the approaches being taken in American Catholic moral theology. Specific questions will be addressed in the chapters which follow.

Birth Issues

Introduction
to
Birth Issues

The medical scientist who reviews the technology of human birth below, Thomas W. Hilgers, M.D., directs the Creighton University Natural Family Planning Education and Research Center. He has done original research in the ovulation method of natural family planning and the "biological valve" which nature provides to assure fresh sperm and ova in the beginning of each new human life.

Dr. William E. May, an associate professor of moral theology at Catholic University where he has been teaching since 1971, presents in his essay a tightly reasoned analysis of human generation as intended by the Creator to occur through marital acts. Dr. May begins with reflections on the role of law in public control of human generation but focuses primarily on the moral norms which flow from the meaning of marriage both as a human covenant and a sacramental mystery.

Rev. Benedict M. Ashley, O.P., a professor of moral theology at Aquinas Institute in Dubuque, Iowa, devotes his attention in "Pro-Life Evangelization" to six groups in the general population who have special interest in and concern for the option of abortion in resolving human value conflicts. His essay synthesizes almost every facet of this agonizing issue which has not lost its moral ugliness despite the permissive legislation and court decisions of recent years.

Professor John T. Noonan, Jr., of the University of California Law School at Berkeley, surveys four great elites which have influenced United States public opinion to tolerate abortion and to overlook the obvious facts of killing human lives. He responds to the political accusations of a single-issue preoccupation among the forces opposing abortion.

These four essays carefully expose the medical, legal, and moral dimensions of the new technology of human birth. The remainder of this volume will turn to human death and the technology for prolonging human life.

The New Technologies of Birth and Death

Thomas W. Hilgers, M.D.

Introduction

Over the past several decades there has been an increasing interest in developing our knowledge of human reproduction. While the reasons for this are many and varied, there are few endeavors which have so attracted the attention of the public. Nearly every type of person, from scientist to lawyer, theologian to politician, has exhibited an interest. With this has come a new technologization of our approach to human reproduction.

It is the purpose of this paper to review the natural state of human reproduction along with its practical application. In addition, how this applies to the new technology and the status of ethically sensitive bio-medical research in this area will also be examined.

I. The Natural Cycle of Human Fertility

Fertility in the human being is cyclic and it is an expression of the *couple*. The fertility potential of the man is, for all practical purposes, continuous from puberty through old age. However, the fertility potential of the woman is naturally cyclic. The woman goes through phases in which she is potentially fertile or infertile. In fact, her potential fertility exists for only a few days in any given menstrual cycle. The exact number of days varies from woman to woman and even within the same woman from cycle to cycle. Of course, neither a man nor a woman is capable of expressing fertility alone. The fertility potentials of the man and the woman must come together at the appropriate times in order for that fertility to be expressed in the creation of a new human life. Therefore, it is fundamental to realize that a proper understanding of human fertility must recognize that it is a combined phenomenon and incapable of being expressed by one individual. In addition, it is naturally cyclic primarily because of the cyclic fertility potential of the woman. Because she is for the most part potentially infertile, the couple is for the most part infertile.

With each ejaculation the male produces, on average, about 400,000,000 sperm.[1] Within each of the normal sperm, there are 23 chromosomes, exactly one-half the number of chromosomes found in all of the other cells in the body. The sperm, then, is a unique cell in the male body. Biologically, the sperm obtain 23 chromosomes by a process of cellular division called *meiosis* which reduces the number of chromosomes to 23. By having only 23 chromosomes (referred to as the *haploid* number of chromosomes) the sperm are ready to be combined with an ovum which also has only 23 chromosomes.

In the conception process, an ovum is combined with a sperm. Why such a large number of sperm are necessary when so few are ultimately used is not entirely understood. However, the sperm are very brittle and fragile cells which have a very difficult time escaping the basically hostile environment of the vagina.

A woman's fertility is expressed biologically in a way which is more complex. The cyclic phases of her fertility are expressed in an understanding of the menstrual cycle. This cycle prepares the woman for the beginning of a new life.

The menstrual cycle begins with the first day of menstrual bleeding and lasts through the last day prior to the beginning of the next menstrual bleeding. The length of this cycle, is, on average, 28 days in duration. However, very few women have 28-day menstrual cycles.[2] The menstrual cycle is irregular in length with wide variations observed in all women. Nonetheless, an understanding of the menstrual cycle is crucial to a proper understanding of the natural cycle of human fertility.

The events in the menstrual cycle are under the control of hormones (chemicals which are produced in one part of the body, travel through the blood stream and effect their action in another part of the body). The primary hormones involved with the menstrual cycle are two hormones produced in the pituitary gland (a pea-sized gland located at the base of the brain) and two hormones produced by the ovary. The follicle-stimulating hormone (FSH) and the luteinizing hormone (LH) are both produced by the pituitary gland.[3,4] FSH stimulates the ovary to produce a *follicle* (a small cyst) which grows and develops on the ovary leading toward ovulation. The ovum is inside the follicle and it undergoes a maturation process as the growth and development process continues. From the initial stimulation of the primary oocyte by FSH until the time of ovulation is about ten days. The first five days result in microscopic changes but the last five days involve macroscopic changes which can be observed with the naked eye. When the follicle has matured sufficiently, the hormone LH surges and results in a rupture of the follicle and release of the ovum. The releasing process is commonly referred to as *ovulation.* Ovulation is one of the critically important events in the menstrual cycle and it is a logical marker (although difficult to detect with precision) with which to divide the menstrual cycle.

During the *pre*ovulatory phase of the menstrual cycle, as the follicle grows and develops, it produces a hormone called *estrogen.* During this phase of the cycle, particularly the last five or six days immediately preceding ovulation, the critical events in the menstrual cycle are under the control of this hormone. Estrogen stimulates the lining cells of the uterus (the endometrium) to grow and to develop. This is a process which has become essential since the previous menstruation sloughed all of these cells. Following menstruation, there is an absolute need for a regeneration of the endometrium if a new human life is ever to be sustained. This rebuilding process in these lining cells is referred to as the *proliferative* phase of the menstrual cycle. As the estrogen levels begin to increase, for the last several days immediately preceding ovulation, this hormone also stimulates the cervix (the opening into the uterus) to produce a characteristic type of cervical mucus which is essential to the adequate function, transport and survivability of the sperm. This mucus is produced in sufficient quantity to literally flow from the cervix, coat the walls of the vagina (thereby neutralizing the acid environment of the vagina) and discharge itself to the opening of the vagina.[5]

As soon as ovulation takes place the tissue on the ovary which had been previously occupied by the follicle now becomes what is called a *corpus luteum* (yellow body). The corpus luteum produces estrogen as does the follicle but now it also produces another hormone called *progesterone*. The progesterone hormone changes the endometrial cells and stimulates their functioning capability. This phase of the menstrual cycle then is referred to as the *secretory phase* primarily because the progesterone hormone stimulates the lining cells of the uterus to secrete an important fluid which is essential to the sustenance of the early human life. The proper functioning of the corpus luteum is essential to the normal expression of our fertility. Not only must the corpus luteum produce adequate amounts of the hormones progesterone and estrogen, but the corpus luteum must also exist for a certain length of time. Ordinarily, the corpus luteum self-destructs 13 days, on average, following ovulation.[6] The self-destruct mechanism is unknown but with it comes a dramatic fall-off in the level of progesterone and estrogen and with the removal of that hormonal support the endometrial cells slough in a process we know as *menstruation*.

The woman is only fertile for a period of time around ovulation. Once the egg is released from the ovary it survives in a state capable of being fertilized for only 12 to 16 hours. However, the couple's fertility is much longer than that in a given menstrual cycle. The one factor which principally dictates the length of the time in which the couple is fertile and infertile in a given menstrual cycle is the cervical mucus. The cervical mucus is produced for a few days, in general, prior to ovulation and is *the vital fluid* which allows for the sperm to, first of all, escape the vagina and, secondly, survive long enough to be available to fertilize the ovum. When the cervical mucus is absent or develops hostile characteristics under hormonal control, such survivability of the sperm does not occur.[3,7,8] This functioning of the cervical mucus could be likened to that of a biological valve.[5,9] The function of this biological valve reflects the natural state of our human fertility and infertility.

It is important to realize that a discussion of the normal functioning of the menstrual cycle and its cyclic phases of fertility and infertility does not alone give a complete picture of the human fertility or infertility potential. Women naturally go through a variety of different reproductive states through the course of their reproductive life. The onset of menstruation in the young girl is referred to as the *menarche.* The cessation of menstruation in an older woman is referred to as the *menopause.* The average age for the menarche is about 13 and the average age for the menopause is about 50.[10] Young girls prior to menarche are generally infertile and women past the menopause are definitely infertile. But from the menarche through menopause there are additional reproductive states in which a woman might find herself.

In the first six to eight years following the menarche and the last six to eight years preceding the menopause, the ovulation process works more sporadically.[2] Women within this time framework are more likely not to ovulate. These women may undergo prolonged periods of *anovulation* in which they are infertile as a result. Similarily, following childbirth, when a woman breastfeeds her child, she may encounter prolonged periods of anovulation secondary to the suppressive effect of the *breastfeeding* itself. Other variations of either anovulation or infrequent ovulation may be observed in the woman coming off the birth control pills, women who are post-partum and not breastfeeding and women who have abnormalities in the hormonal functioning of their systems. For an adequate understanding of the fertility phases in the human it is essential that adequate account be taken of these natural states of reproductive quiescence.

Finally, it is essential to realize that the whole mechanism of the fertility process is highly sophisticated and very finely tuned. When the process is disturbed for one reason or another, a disruption in function may result. Ultimately, a continued growth in our understanding of the natural cycle of human fertility should not only allow us to achieve and avoid pregnancy naturally but also be of assistance in the remedy of some serious reproductive anomalies.

II. The Beginning of Human Life

After ovulation occurs, the ovum is taken up by the fallopian tube and moves down toward the cavity of the uterus. This movement takes place because the peristaltic action of the tube is in that direction and because of the presence of microscopic, hairlike projections, called cilia, which rhythmically beat also in that direction.[1]

If sperm are deposited in the vagina when the "good" cervical muscus is present around the time of ovulation, some of the sperm will escape the vagina, migrate through the cervix and go to the fallopian tubes where they encounter the fresh ovum. The sperm move primarily as the result of the beating action of their tails. In the presence of good cervical mucus, sperm have been detected in the fallopian tubes within five minutes after their placement in the vagina.[11]

In many animal species a process referred to as *capacitation* is known to occur. This is a metabolic and enzymatic change which the sperm must necessarily undergo in order to be capable of fertilizing the egg. It has been thought that the process of capacitation of the sperm occurs as the sperm travel through the female reproductive tract. While it has been speculated that such a capacitation process occurs in the human, there is as yet no convincing evidence to prove or disprove it.

The ovum has an outer layer called the *zona pellucida.* This membrane is of vital importance. In its own way, it acts as a shell for the egg. As sperm approach the ovum, the zona acts to assure that only one sperm penetrates and enters the cellular matter of the ovum. When the sperm has penetrated the ovum, there exists for a short period of time two *pronuclei.* The 23-chromosome package of the sperm is separate from the 23-chromosome package of the ovum. When the two pronuclei fuse, the biologic qualities of an individual human life come into existence. This process is usually referred to as *fertilization or conception.* Surely, the fusion of the pronuclei occurs within minutes to hours after the penetration of the sperm into the cytoplasm of the ovum.

Once conception has occurred, an individual human life has come into existence[12-23] and is a progressive, ongoing continuum until natural or artifically induced death ensues. This is a fact so well established within the reproductive sciences that no intellectually honest physician in full command of modern knowledge could dare to deny it. There is no authority in medicine or biology who can be cited to refute this concept.

Immediately following conception, the single cell within the zona pellucida is called the *zygote*. Within 24 hours the zygote begins to divide into 2, 4, 8, 16, etc., cells. While this is occurring, the new human life moves down the fallopian tube towards the uterus. The hormones progesterone and estrogen are increasing their levels preparing the lining of the uterus. At this stage, the solid mass of cells is called a *morula*. As cellular division continues, a fluid-filled cavity appears in the morula. At this stage, it is called a *blastocyst*. It takes approximately 6 days for the new human life to make its way to the uterus. At that time, it is in the blastocyst stage of development.

The blastocyst divides into an *inner* and an *outer* cell mass. The inner cell mass is the early differentiation of the embryo and the outer cell mass is the early differentiation of the supportive structures, the placenta and membranes. These structures then are uniquely created by the newly conceived individual for his or her ultimate survival.

As the blastocyst enters the uterus, the lining cells have been prepared to nurture the new life. In all of its early development, the actual volume of the blastocyst is no larger at this stage than the original ovum. The zona pellucida now ruptures and the blastocyst attaches itself to the wall of the uterus where it burrows into the cellular structure making a maternal-embryological connection. This process is referred to as *implantation* or *nidation*. From this point forward the growth and development of the embryo (up to 8 weeks) and fetus (after 8 weeks) is taken up within the uterus.

Many have placed great value on the nidational process saying that it is *the* key event in the developmental process. They would argue that implantation is *essential* to ongoing growth and development and without it, one experiences an unnoticed pre-implantation loss. Add to this the often repeated notion that the natural pre-implantation loss is very high, and the nidation event has taken on additional meaning and emphasis.[9] In addition, questions of twinning and recombination, which conditions are said to be complete only by the time of implantation, and the fact that so many modern "contraceptives" work in the perinidational period, all have lent a certain force to this recent emphasis.

No one could argue that implantation is a minor event. Indeed, it is ultimately an *essential* ingredient to the *continued development* of the newly conceived human. However, the *ultimate* essential ingredient to all of human life's processes is *the conception event* itself. Surely birth is as essential as implantation but both depend ultimately upon conception. There is *no* biologic reason to place implantation or birth at a higher level of order or value than conception. However, since conception precedes these latter events and is *essential* to the *very potential* of their occurrence, it surely would be of a higher order of value. Simple common sense dictates this. The arguments mentioned previously will be dealt with in greater detail later.

Twins occur about once in 90 births. Two of every three sets of twins are fraternal or nonidentical twins. Fraternal twins result when the ovary ovulates two eggs and they are both fertilized although by separate sperm. Identical twins, occurring once in 270 births, result from the early division of a zygote or early morula into two "identical" cell masses with subsequent development from that point forward. It is currently thought that such a cleavage occurs very early, within 24-48 hours after conception, and that there is a high likelihood that it is a genetically predetermined phenomenon and not simply a spontaneous event.[24]

From conception, the child is a complex, dynamic, rapidly growing individual. By a natural and continuous process the single-cell zygote will, over approximately nine months, develop into the trillions of cells of the newborn. The natural end of the sperm and the ovum is death unless fertilization occurs. Or, to say it another way, we are neither grown-up sperm nor are we grown-up eggs. At fertilization a new and unique individual is created which, although receiving its chromosomes from each parent, is really unlike either.[25-28]

III. Achieving and Avoiding Pregnancy – The Science and Art of Natural Family Planning

Throughout the centuries, most couples have had little difficulty achieving pregnancy. Knowledge of exactly how or when pregnancy was achieved was another matter. To know how to avoid pregnancy without complete avoidance of genital contact was generally unheard of. The ability to know and understand the phases of fertility and infertility in a way which can be put into practical use is a modern development and has become known as *natural family planning*.

Such systems of understanding were not available prior to 1929 and 1930. In those years, Knaus[29] in Austria and Ogino[30] in Japan independently discovered that ovulation occurred about 14 days before the next period. This important discovery settled the issue of when ovulation occurred. It laid the groundwork for the development of natural family planning.

The initial history of natural family planning (NFP) focused on the identification of the days of infertility only. Originally, calendar calculations were used and later the shift in the basal body temperature. The latter identified that ovulation had passed and that infertility was therefore present. The identification of the time of fertility was for the most part accomplished, until recently, by subtraction. A more precise understanding of *both* the phases of fertility *as well as* the phases of infertility is essential to a true understanding of natural family planning.

Over the years, research into NFP has been plagued by the predilection for identifying ovulation, so-called ovulation detection. In recent years, the emphasis has been on *fertility detection* and this is much more practical. In addition, much time has been spent on discussing signs which, of and by themselves, have had nothing to do with our fertility. Such signs as mittelschmerz ("mid-cycle" pain), breast tenderness, vulvar swelling, abdominal bloating, intermenstrual bleeding, changes in the cervix (cephalad shift, dilation and softening) and basal body temperature changes are themselves *secondary signs* which have no *direct* bearing on the expression of our fertility. With the focus of the past 10 years on cervical mucus discharge, NFP has begun to deal with a sign which is itself *essential* to our fertility. It is this cervical mucus which accounts for sperm survival and penetration through the cervix. Indeed, it is this cervical mucus which dictates the length of the time of fertility. Knowledge of the discharge has brought a challenging new balance into our thinking of NFP. Indeed it has allowed for a much more precise identification of the time of fertility without losing precision to identify the time of infertility.

There are several methods of natural family planning. All of these methods depend upon the complete avoidance of genital contact during the time of fertility if the methods are to be used successfully to avoid pregnancy. All of these methods are shared methods, involving the cooperation of both husband and wife. They vary mostly in the precision with which they identify the phases of fertility and infertility and in their overall applicability to women of different reproductive categories. The following is a brief description of these methods.

The Calendar Method: In this method, calculations are obtained by the use of past cycle history (6-12 months), theoretical ovum and sperm survival times, and the presupposed time from ovulation to menstruation. By putting this information into a formula, a time of pre- and post-ovulatory infertility is obtained. Generally, the method requires regular cycles and is useless to the 20-30% of women who may not be in such cycles.

This method has become known as the Calendar *Rhythm* Method. The calculations used to define post-ovulatory infertility in this method are no longer used. However, some form of calendar calculation for the identification of pre-ovulatory infertility is still in widespread practice. Overall, the precision of the methodology is low.[41]

The Basal Body Temperature (BBT) Method: This method was first described by Father Wilhelm Hillebrand, a German Catholic priest, in 1934.[2] It is a post-ovulatory method only. When a woman takes and records her basal body temperature daily she will detect a rise in the temperature to a new, higher level after ovulation has passed. The rise in temperature is due to the thermogenic properties of the hormone progesterone. Once the temperature sustains the higher level for three days, the time of post-ovulatory infertility is said to have begun.[31]

Overall, this method is restrictive since it limits intercourse to the post-ovulatory time only. In addition, it is of no help in identifying a time of fertility. Also, when used by itself, the BBT is wrong about 5% of the time in correctly identifying post-ovulation infertility.[32] Furthermore, it is useless in the woman with prolonged anovulation (e.g. the breast-feeding mother).

The Calendar-Thermic Method: Recognizing the restrictiveness of the BBT Method, investigators have combined calculation for identification of a time of pre-ovulatory infertility with the shift in the BBT curve. Their are several different types of calendar calculations which have been described. Roetzer,[33] Vollman,[34] Doring,[35] Marshall,[31,36] and Kippley[43] have all described different versions. While the combination effectively decreases the amount of avoidance of genital contact, it maintains the same problems as either one used alone. It is imprecise at identifying the time of fertility and useless in women with prolonged anovulation.

The Sympto-Thermic Method: The Sympto-Thermic Method is a post-ovulatory method only. By combining the woman's observation of the PEAK symptom[38] (see below) with the shift in BBT, and waiting for at least three full days of BBT shift to occur *past the PEAK,* the time of post-ovulatory infertility is identified. By combining the two signs, the deficiencies which are inherent in the BBT alone are overcome.[32] However, adding BBT measurements to the PEAK symptom observation is unnecessary and is less precise.[32]

In order to obtain a time of defined pre-ovulatory infertility with the Sympto-Thermic Method, a calendar calculation is added (the Calendar-Sympto-Thermic Method) or Ovulation Method instructions (see below) are utilized. Again, because the methodology focuses on the BBT shift, it cannot be applied in those circumstances where ovulation is suspended.

The Ovulation Method: The newest method of NFP is called the Ovulation Method. The Ovulation Method is based upon the woman's observation of a characteristic discharge of cervical mucus. This mucus begins *prior* to ovulation and reflects the ovaries' pre-ovulatory production of estrogen. The method is more precise in its identification of the times of fertility and infertility than any other natural method. In addition, it gives the couple positive information not only on the time of infertility but also the time of fertility. It has removed the idea of "taking a chance" and it provides couples with positive information on when they can achieve a pregnancy.

The method is an *estrogen dependent method* unlike the BBT methods which are *progesterone dependent.* In other words, the presence of the mucus symptom is *not* dependent upon the formation of a corpus luteum (which only occurs after ovulation) but rather upon follicular development (which is the process leading up to ovulation). As a result, it is a method which can be used at any stage of a woman's reproductive life. The prolonged absence of ovulation is reflected in the general pattern of a prolonged absence of mucus discharge. When follicular development begins, estrogen is produced and the characteristic mucus appears.

Effectiveness: When discussing the effectiveness of natural methods of family planning we *must* keep in mind the fact that these methods can be used as methods of achieving pregnancy as well as methods of avoiding pregnancy. In discussing overall effectiveness, it is *essential* that this overall perspective be kept; otherwise we find ourselves concerned with their contraceptive effectiveness only. This becomes very important when comparing the Ovulation Method with BBT-based methodologies.

In both cases, when the methods are used according to instruction as methods of avoiding pregnancy, the method effectiveness is in the 99+ percentile of effectiveness. *At this time, no survey has yet been undertaken which properly evaluates these methods as methods of achieving a pregnancy.* The reason for this can be found in the historical development of statistical protocols used for such purposes. These protocols were developed with contraceptives *only* in mind. They were *not* developed with NFP in mind. Often intimidated by the charge that NFP needs to be subjected to the same scientific scrutiny as other contraceptives, even NFP investigators have until now focused only on contraceptive effectiveness. Because of this, there has been an ongoing debate regarding effectiveness which will not be resolved until proper protocols are developed. This will take several years yet before a final answer.[39]

Delivery of Service: It should be stated *ever so emphatically* that NFP is *practical, useable and deliverable* to people. For those who might object to the concept of genital avoidance, this is not the problem it is made out to be. In fact, it has been observed as promotive of non-genital communication within the relationship. However, a *great deal* needs to be done in establishing delivery systems.

There are several misunderstandings which need to be corrected relating to service delivery. It is important that these misunderstandings be corrected since often important administrative decisions related to NFP delivery are made by individuals who *do not have* adequate background in NFP itself. The following are very important to understand:

1. The actual *use* of a natural method is really relatively easy. While definite problems in use can be identified, and no one wishes to overstate the case, these can usually be corrected and improvements in this area are developing rapidly.

2. *Teaching* natural family planning is *not easy.* Natural family planning is best delivered by teachers who are *well trained* and are *themselves users.* The emphasis here is on "well trained" because it is in this area where the greatest recognition of need is required. The NFP teacher must know how to effectively teach *any* person who requests these services. This requires teaching skills, knowledge of all phases of reproductive biology, knowledge of problem recognition and problem solving. Such training *cannot* occur in a weekend or over short

periods of time. If such approaches are taken, the quality of service will be significantly reduced. We must develop a sense of seriousness about the training of NFP teachers and be willing to expend the time, energy and money to develop well-trained teachers.[40]

3. We must begin to understand that the *well-trained* NFP teacher is a *professional person* obtaining his or her professional standing from the highly responsible and relatively sensitive nature of the work. This professionalism will grow as the teachers gain in experience working with the dynamics of couples who know and understand their fertility.

4. Finally, within the above contexts, it is *very important* to realize that we are at *the beginning* of our work in NFP, not the end. The next five to ten years could be very exciting if we make good decisions now. Ultimately we have a very important challenge before us as Catholics. We *must* develop a delivery system for *quality* NFP services which is available to *everyone* in the Catholic community. While such program development should *not* in any way be limited to Catholics, at the same time, the Catholic population *must* have access to these services. The challenge of *Humanae Vitae*[41] is already 12 years old and we all are very late. The Church and its people can live by *Humanae Vitae,* but it is critical that *the will* of the Church to do so *be developed and exhibited.*

Future Research Needs: It seems important to point out, probably because there appears to be so little public identification of the fact, that it is *amazing* just how little research has been done in the area of natural family planning in the last 50 years. If one were to compare the amount of research effort and research dollars that have been put into NFP versus contraceptive and abortion development, the percentage would be *far less than one percent.* The development of NFP over the years has come about because of the supreme dedication, out of faith, of a handful of Catholic doctors and lay people. Now, as development is increasing, the number of people involved also is increasing. However, the initial work was done by just a few.

This is said in part to shame all of us who have not contributed although wondering why the Church teaches as it does. On the other hand, it is also said simply to point out how much more needs to be done.

Through research, method-related problems can be solved, basic physiologic correlations can be made, effectiveness studies can be properly designed and carried out, etc. Through research an exciting agenda for understanding the behavioral dimensions of NFP use can develop and such behavioral patterns can be more clearly defined and understood. It is through research that we can test educational curricula for our NFP teachers so that improvements and refinements can be made.

IV. Artificial Reproduction

As the new technology "advances" there is a clear trend toward reproduction's becoming more and more artificial. Such issues as artificial insemination, *in vitro* fertilization, cloning, the development of artificial wombs, cross-genetic breeding, etc., are all vehicles of a brave new world. But the brave new world is no longer in the future. The first two items on this list are currently available for use in man: cloning has been accomplished in animals and artificial wombs are in the research stages. This discussion will focus only on artificial insemination, *in vitro* fertilization and cloning.

Artificial Insemination: There are two basic forms of artificial insemination: homologous artificial insemination (AIH) and artificial insemination donor (AID).[42] In the first instance, the woman's husband is the source of the seminal fluid, whereas in the second instance an unknown male donor is the source of the sperm and seminal fluid. In both procedures, the seminal fluid is obtained by masturbation. Sometimes the sperm and seminal fluid are frozen for storage purposes prior to the actual insemination procedure. However, most people in this field would wish to use fresh seminal fluid. With both procedures, the seminal fluid is placed into a syringe which is attached to a long cannula which is in turn placed against the cervix and a small amount of seminal fluid is placed against the external cervical canal. This insemination procedure is carried out around the time of ovulation as estimated by clinical parameters. From a purely medical point of view, there appears to be no advantage to the use of homologous artificial insemination. Artificially placing the seminal fluid into the vagina cannot be proven as any better than natural insemination. However, the psychological risks that are played with in this procedure relate to a professional reinforcement of male incompetence. The physician is saying to the male partner that he is inadequate to properly inseminate his wife whereas the physician, with his technology, can do the job better. This leaves the male with serious questions about his fertility. Unfortunately, there is very little opportunity for the husband to even ventilate his feelings in this regard. I have found in my own practice, in dealing with couples who have been artificially inseminated by other physicians, that the husband finds the repetitive masturbating highly unsatisfactory and degrading.

With donor insemination, the seminal fluid is obtained from a male who is paid to masturbate and donate his seminal fluid. The donor signs a release so that all legal attachments are severed. Since many of the donor insemination programs are associated with medical schools, one of the most commonly used resources for seminal fluid are male medical students. To some of these individuals, donating their seminal fluid for the eventual conception of countless numbers of unknown children seems to be some form of ego trip. The desire of the physicians involved in the insemination process to hire medical students for the production of "high quality" spermatozoa seems to be a bit arrogant to say the least. Donor insemination is fraught with potential psychological and legal complications. For the husband who must passively participate in this insemination process, serious feelings of guilt may arise. Again, no opportunity for ventilation of these feelings is available. The general attitude is that the male "is tough" and can put up with this without it causing any difficulties.

In addition to the potential psychological and legal problems which are associated with donor insemination, one cannot help but be struck by the basic dishonesty of the procedure. For example, it is not uncommon for the physician to recommend that the husband and wife have intercourse on the day in which the artificial donor insemination has taken place. In this way, nobody will ever know whether it was the husband's sperm or the donor's sperm which was responsible for the conception. It has even been recommended that the woman be delivered by an obstetrician who is unaware of the method of insemination, so that he can sign the birth certificate without committing perjury.[42] The blanket of secrecy which covers AID raises many serious questions.

In Vitro Fertilization: On July 25, 1978, baby Louise Brown was born in England as the result of an *in vitro* (in glass) fertilization procedure and embryo transfer. This was the first report which has been reasonably credible regarding the successful gestation of an *in vitro* fertilization procedure. However, the procedure utilized in that case has only been presented at clinical meetings and to the date of this writing has not been fully published. The only written report was a brief letter to the editor of *The Lancet* on August 12, 1978, written by the principals involved, Steptoe and Edwards.[43]

In vitro fertilization has also been referred to as "the test tube baby." The ovum is obtained from the ovary by means of aspiration of the follicle around the time of ovulation through the laparoscope. Usually, the ovary is stimulated by medications to progress toward ovulation under artificial stimulation. The reason for this is to improve the timing of ovum retrieval. Once the ovum is obtained, it is placed into a nutritive medium, and sperm, obtained by masturbation from either the husband or a donor, is mixed with the ovum. The two are then allowed to join and the early growth and development of the embryo is witnessed in the petri dish. When the early morula reaches the 8-cell stage it is then transferred into the uterine cavity for continued growth and development. Nobody knows for sure how many conceptions occur for every successful implantation. However, the overwhelming majority of early morulae would die because of unsuccessful implantation. *In vitro* fertilization is not a new concept. In 1944, Rock and Menkin[44] reported in *Science* magazine that they had isolated more than 800 human follicular eggs from surgical material and that 138 of these were observed after exposure to sperm that were washed in Locke's solution. The eggs were usually cultured in fresh human serum. After 22 to 27 hours, two eggs were described as being in the 2-cell stage and two in the 3-cell stage. In 1963, Hayashi,[45] in Japan, collected 160 ova from 74 patients and cultured them in a basic salt solution and human serum with gonadotropins and various steroids added. While he claims to have obtained cleavage in 20 eggs, critical evaluation of his illustrations of fertilized and cleaving eggs by Blandau revealed that they were not fertilized and segmenting ova but rather fragmenting ova (which are unfertilized).[46] Steptoe and Edwards began publishing their work on *in vitro* fertilization in 1966. Between 1966 and 1970, 473 eggs were inseminated in a variety of media with a fertilization rate ranging from 1.6 to 42.0%.[47-50] In 1976, Steptoe and Edwards first reported successful reimplantation of a human embryo which subsequently developed into a tubal pregnancy.[51] It was impossible to determine from their publication precisely how many embryo transfers were carried out unsuccessfully before this report. Bevis in 1974 reported in the *British Medical Journal* the birth of three children who were "apparently normal, were alive in the United Kingdom in Western Europe after embryo implantation."[52] The details of these transplant patients have never appeared in the world's literature. And finally, on December 25, 1978, the *Medical World News* published a report that doctors Mukherjee and Bhattacharya, in India, had sucessfully undertaken an *in vitro* fertilization with embryo transfer and successful birth of a baby girl. However, there has been no official documentation or verification that this, in fact, happened. On August 12, 1978, in a letter to the editor of *Lancet,* Steptoe and Edwards[43] reported the birth of an infant girl weighing 2700 grams. "Pregnancy was established after laparoscopic recovery of an oocyte on November 10, 1977, *in vitro* fertilization and normal cleavage in culture media, and the reimplantation of the 8 cell embryo into the uterus 2½ days later." While this description has been amplified at several clinical meetings it has not yet been published so that it can be scientifically scrutinized.

Blandau, in a recent review of this subject,[46] points out some of the difficulties in analyzing the *in vitro* fertilization data: "Attempts to summarize the results of *in vitro* fertilization of human oocytes from the world's literature can be a most frustrating experience. Frequently there is no indication of the total number of eggs recovered in comparison to the number of oocytes inseminated. There often are no data on the number of patients from which the eggs have been collected, the state of their menstrual cycles, or whether or not they have been treated to induce follicular growth and ovum maturation. The criteria for fertilization and segmentation are not adequately documented. The figures published to illustrate fertilization and segmentation either are of poor quality or reveal significant abnormalities, particularly cellular vesiculation or fragmentation. Much needs to be done in this key area to present more accurate and convincing evidence. The tools for accomplishing this are available."

In vitro fertilization has been promoted as a possible solution to those women whose infertility problem is related to an irreversible and untreatable form of tubal obstruction. There are, of course, millions of women in the world with such a problem and having this technology available would serve a great demand. There is little question that the procedure causes extensive waste of preimplantation human embryos. This has created a considerable amount of controversy. *In vitro* fertilization has been a controversial issue, however, since at least 1970 when laboratory fertilization of human ova with human sperm became much more technically feasible. In 1975, the Department of Health, Education, and Welfare declared a moratorium on federal funding of *in vitro* fertilization until an ethics board had met and made recommendations to the HEW Secretary. An HEW Ethics Advisory Board was formed in 1978. The board's inquiry was prompted by the petition for funding of *in vitro* research by Dr. Pierre Soupart of Vanderbilt University. The Ethics Advisory Board, however, widened its scope to include the ethics of clinical (where embryos are implanted into infertile women) as well as research application (where embryos are created solely for research purposes).

On September 15, 1978 the Ethics Advisory Board began public hearings on *in vitro* fertilization and issued its report on June 18, 1979. In that report, the advisory board concluded that *in vitro* fertilization, both in clinical and research contexts, is "acceptable from an ethical standpoint." This was a unanimously accepted position and included the support of some very notable Catholic moral theologians in the United States. This board did not rule specifically on Dr. Soupart's proposal but suggested that it be reviewed again in light of their report. Public input into the Department of HEW was extended from August 17, 1979 through January 8, 1980 by the new Secretary of HEW, Patricia Harris. The decision as to whether or not to fund the Soupart proposal is to be made sometime after the new public input closes.

Cloning: There has been some recent publicity given to the subject of cloning. The book *In His Image: The Cloning of Man,* by freelance writer David Rorvik, caused considerable controversy a couple of years ago. Claiming that a millionaire recluse of a man had funded the first successful cloning procedure, it created a considerable amount of Orwellian discussion. However, no verification or documentation that this has been accomplished was ever put forth. In fact, most of the scientists who might be near such potential capability stated emphatically that such could not possibly have occurred given our current scientific understanding.

This notwithstanding, a brief description of cloning seems appropriate. *Cloning* is also known as nuclear transplantation. The concept is a reasonably simple one. The nucleus of the fresh ovum is dissected out utilizing a special dissecting microscope. Another cell from within the adult body, referred to as a *somatic* cell, is also denucleated. The nucleus from the somatic cell is then transplanted into the ovum. When this occurs, the potential exists for the complete replication of an individual genetically identical to the donor of the somatic nucleus. The egg, discovering that it has a full set of chromosomes instead of the half-set found in unfertilized ova, responds by beginning to divide as if it had been normally fertilized. This has been accomplished in frogs.

This form of asexual reproduction would allow man to reproduce himself, creating virtually genetically identical human beings. Thus, the future could offer such phenomena as a police force cloned from the cells of J. Edgar Hoover, an invincible basketball team cloned from Kareem Abdul Jabbar, or perhaps the colonization of the moon by astronauts cloned from a "genetically sound" specimen chosen by NASA officials. Using the same technique, a woman could even have a child cloned from one of her own cells. The child would inherit all its mother's characteristics including, of course, her sex.

Dramatic as cloning may be, it may be overshadowed in temporal significance by a technique that may well be practiced before the end of this century: genetic surgery, or correction of man's "inherited imperfections" at the level of the genes themselves. When molecular biologists learn to map the location of specific genes in human DNA strands, determine the genetic code of each and then create synthetic genes in the test tube, they will have the ability to perform genetic surgery.

Some molecular biologists envisage using laser beams to slice through DNA molecules at desired points, burning out faulty genes. These would then be replaced by segments of DNA tailored in the test tube to emulate a properly functioning gene and introduced into the body as artificial viruses. This could have potentially beneficial effects in the treatment of various disease processes. However, if used inappropriately, it could have far ranging devastating effects.

It should be pointed out that it is not the expressed intention of this paper to discuss the ethical aspects of artificial insemination, *in vitro* fertilization and cloning. However, it should be known that the author feels that very strong arguments can be made against those procedures. Those procedures should be viewed as being intrinsically unhealthy to mind, body *and* spirit.

V. Perinidational Abortion

Much of the thrust in "contraceptive" development in the past twenty years has been aimed at the destruction of the life of the early blastocyst just prior to, at the time of, and shortly after implantation. This perinidational period of time is currently the most frequently attacked period of pregnancy. Clearly, more abortions are artificially induced during this period of time than at any time later in the pregnancy. The major thrust of "contraceptive" research in the United States today is in *perinidational abortion.*

There are several agents which require discussion in this section. The most obvious will be the intrauterine devices. However, coming under this heading will be a discussion of oral "contraceptives," "morning after" pills, prostaglandins and menstrual extraction.

There are basically three types of intrauterine device (IUD) designs which are in common usage today. While these three designs have much in common regarding their mechanism of action, there are enough differences to warrant separate consideration.

Polyethylene Devices: It is certain that the polyethylene devices provoke a myriad of unnatural effects on the female reproductive system. These effects, working in unison, undoubtedly contribute to their ultimate action. That these IUDs do not interfere significantly with the menstrual cycle, ovulation or sperm migration appears well settled. There seems to be little question that active sperm, in adequate numbers, do reach the fallopian tubes, where fertilization normally takes place. No evidence at the present time suggests that fertilization itself is prevented consistently. On the contrary, the evidence supports the concept that fertilization occurs at normal or near normal frequency.[53]

Present knowledge indicates that the mechanism of action of the IUD on the endometrium, myometrial activity, and the intrauterine biochemical and biological milieu is destructive in nature; under these conditions, the blastocyst is unable to survive. A complete and detailed review of studies done on humans can be found elsewhere.[53]

The view that the IUD destroys the blastocyst is now almost universally accepted.[54,58] Recent work with the radioreceptorassay and the radioimmunoassay for Human Chorionic Gonadotropin (HCG) clearly supports this concept.[56] These sophisticated pregnancy tests are capable of detecting pregnancy 6-10 days after conception, or shortly after implantation. The production of the pregnancy hormone

HCG is dependent upon implantation; therefore, the detection of its production prior to the onset of menses in IUD users suggests that the IUD disrupts the blastocyst *after* implantation.

Copper-clad Devices: Some intrauterine devices are made of polyethylene in the shape of a "T" or a "7" with a small copper wire wound around the core of the IUD. The copper wire which is incorporated into these devices is slowly dissolved over a period of time at a rate of 50-75 micrograms per day.[57] The effectiveness of the devices slowly deteriorates because of the loss of copper; therefore a change in the device is recommended every four years.[54] Without the addition of copper, the "T" and "7" designs are very ineffective.[57] As a result, the copper plays a role in the birth control effectiveness of these devices. It has been shown that a surface area of copper at 200 mm^2 in size is necessary to effect its action.[58]

It appears that copper has little effect on sperm motility in *utero.*[59] It has also been shown that when copper IUDs are inserted post-coitally they are effective in preventing continuing pregnancy.[59,60] This has been a proposed treatment for the woman who is the victim of sexual assault. It seems that this result could only be accomplished if implantation were disrupted.

While the effects of intrauterine copper are at this time not fully understood, it appears safe to say that it acts in a multitude of ways which result in disruption of the blastocysts.

Progesterone Devices: Shaped in the form of a "T", these devices have progesterone in the vertical core. The progesterone devices contain enough hormone to last approximately one year.[61] It has been shown that the small amount of hormone released does not consistently block ovulation.[62] While the progesterone may affect the cervical mucus, sperm "capacitation," and sperm metabolism,[63] it is generally thought that the primary mechanism is related to progesterone-produced local changes in the endometrium which render it incapable of sustaining implantation.[54,61,63]

The intrauterine devices act at the uterine level by destroying the blastocysts. In addition, if implantation occurs and continuing pregnancy is established, one can expect a much higher incidence of spontaneous abortion.[53] For the individual couple it is important that they be aware of this information so that they may make an informed ethical and moral decision regarding the use of an IUD. Far too often, the woman is told by her physician that its mechanism of action is unknown. For the physician, it is no longer adequate to make that claim. In the 1960's the mechanism may not have been clear; however, in the 1970's it is all too clear. On May 10, 1977, the Food and Drug Administration issued their text of required patient information for IUDs. [64] In it they wrote that "IUD's seem to interfere in some manner with the implantation of the fertilized egg in the lining of the uterine cavity. The IUD does not prevent ovulation."

With the oral "contraceptives" there has been a greater resistance to labeling them as either abortifacient or potentially so. When the oral "contraceptive" first came on the market in the early 1960's, the major thrust of its mechanism of action was said to be a suppressive effect on ovulation. By creating an anovulatory condition, these new pills would truly be contraceptive by preventing the sperm from reaching the ovum. However, the birth control pills which are currently on the market are not the same chemically as those birth control pills which came on the market originally.

The standard birth control pill contains a synthetic progesterone-like hormone and a synthetic estrogen-like hormone in combination. The major difference between the pills of 1960 and the pills of 1980 is in the dosage of estrogen contained in the pill. Today's pills have much less estrogen in them than their ancestors. It is the estrogen-like hormone which is primarily responsible for the suppression of ovulation. With the amount of this hormone reduced in the contemporary birth control pills, the incidence of "escape ovulation" has increased. As a result, ovulation may occur as often as 25% to 30% of the time in women using the newer birth control pills. [65]

The manufacturers of the oral "contraceptives" are required to put the following description of their mechanism of action in the package inserts: "Combination oral contraceptives act primarily through the mechanism of gonadatrophin suppression due to the estrogenic and progestational activity of the ingredients. Although the primary mechanism of action is inhibition of ovulation, alterations in the genital tract include changes in the cervical mucus (which increase the difficulty of sperm penetration) and the endometrium (which reduce the likelihood of implantation) and may also contribute to contraceptive effectiveness." [66] How often the anti-nidational effect of the birth control pills is actually called upon is not known. However, clearly the potential for that exists and hardly anyone would deny that, at the very least, this may occur occasionally.

Another type of birth control pill is called the "mini-pill." These pills contain no estrogen and only progesterone-like compounds. The required labelling is as follows: "The primary mechanism through which (name of pill) prevents conception is not known, but progestin-only contraceptives are known to alter the cervical mucus, exert a progestational effect on the endometrium, interfering with implantation and, in some patients, suppress ovulation."[67]

The so-called "morning after" pill is an estrogen-like hormone, usually Diethylstilbesterol (DES). These hormones are most commonly prescribed to the victim of sexual assault. The evidence would suggest at the present time that the use of these hormones in this fashion should be considered abortifacient.

Prostaglandins are compounds which are found in nearly every bodily fluid. In addition, they have many different effects. Prostaglandin research, because of the wide-spread potential use of these compounds, is a field of and by itself. However, the early research with prostaglandins has gone into their abortifacient capability. In the area of perinidational abortion prostaglandins, vaginal suppositories are currently being developed. These suppositories are given on a monthly basis to assist in the establishment of menstruation. By "bringing on a period" the woman would not know if she were pregnant or not. Clearly, the intent in the use of the prostaglandins in this fashion would be to disrupt implantation. While such suppositories are currently in only the research stages, it is thought that they might be commercially available within the next three to five years.

Finally, menstrual extraction or menstrual regulation is becoming more and more practiced in the United States. Menstrual extraction is accomplished by inserting a small polyethylene catheter into the uterus through the cervix and, with suction, the catheter is then withdrawn. This process physically disrupts the endometrium and creates an abortion if the woman is pregnant. Such menstrual extractions are recommended to be performed within the first one to two weeks following the first missed menstrual period. As an alternative, the procedure may be performed on a monthly basis, as with the prostaglandin suppositories, at the time of the expected menstrual period. In both of these cases, the abortion would be performed in the very early stages post-implantation. In many such cases, the woman may not be pregnant when the procedure is performed.

VI. The Status of Ethically Sensitive Biomedical Research

In the past 40 years there has been an exponential growth in the amount of biomedical research which has gone into the area of human reproduction. If one were to do an evaluation of *private and public funding* sources that have gone into this sector of the research community, one would find an exponential growth in dollars especially during the 1950's and 1960's. There has been some leveling off in the 70's although there continues to be an increase. *Almost universally,* the funds have gone toward research in contraception, perinidational abortion, and abortion itself. There has been some limited funding of basic research in human reproduction, but nearly all of this has been stimulated from private and governmental interest in the "newer, safer, better, improved contraceptive or abortifacient." Even research into infertility has received a low priority in the last twenty or thirty years.

In looking at the changes in abortion policies in this country in the past ten years, nearly all of the debates, including Justice Blackmun's famous decision, *Roe v. Wade,*[68] include strong support of evidence supplied by the scientific community in favor of abortion and contraception. There has been very little, if any, scientific support presented for what could be called the pro-life position.

The lack of substantial scientific research in human reproduction from a pro-life point of view exists for several reasons. Clearly, there has been no substantive funding available, especially from the government but also from private sources, to conduct such research. Secondly, there have not been sufficient investigative interests on the part of pro-life investigators to involve themselves in research of this nature. Thirdly, availability of a research population has been limited.

In short, the amount of research which has gone into the study of human reproduction which is pro-life in its orientation has been almost nonexistent. In fact, the scarcity of research is appalling. In a society in which laws or policies tend not to change without "scientific proof," the movement to respect life must develop strongly in the area of research in human reproduction. *This research can be done ethically and totally pro-life. No compromises need to be made.* What will be needed, of course, will be sufficient funding and, ultimately, the people with skill and aptitude who are willing to approach these problems out of a sense of true obligation and responsibility and within the framework of a very sensitive and privileged respect for human life.

References

1. Hartman, CG: Science and the Safe Period. Williams and Wilkins, Baltimore, 1962.
2. Vollman, R: The Menstrual Cycle. WB Saunders, Philadelphia, 1977.
3. Moghissi, KS, Syner, FN, Evans, TN: A complete picture of the menstrual cycle. Am J Obstet Gynecol 114:405, 1972.
4. Punnonen, R, Nummi, S, Ylikorkals, O, et al: A composite picture of the normal menstrual cycle. Act Obstet Gynecol Scand (Suppl) 51:64, 1975.
5. Hilgers, TW and Prebil, AM: The Ovulation Method – Vulvar Observations as an index of Fertility/Infertility. Obstet Gynec 53:12, 1979.
6. Hilgers, TW: The Length of the Luteal Phase (in press).
7. Kroeks, MVAM, and Kremer, J: The influence of coitus and alkalinizing irrigation on pH in cervical mucus and vaginal contents (abstract). Fertil Steril 28:387, 1977.
8. Jaszcak, S, and Hafez, ESE: Pathophysiology of human vaginal fluid in infertility work-up (abstract). Fertil Steril 28:387, 1977.
9. Hilgers, TW: Human Reproduction – Three Issues for the Moral Theologian. Theological Studies, 38:136, 1977.
10. Treloar, AA: Variations in the Human Menstrual Cycle. In: Proceedings of a Research Conference on Natural Family Planning, The Human Life Foundation, 1972.
11. Davajan, V, Nakamura, R and Kharma, K: Spermatoza Transport in Cervical Mucus. Obstet Gynec Survey 25:1, 1970.
12. Patten, BM: Human Embryology, 3d ed. McGraw-Hill, NY, 1968, pp. 41-43.
13. Arey, CB: Developmental Anatomy: A Textbook and Laboratory Manual of Embryology. WB Saunders, Philadelphia and London, 1965, p. 55.
14. Langmann, J: Medical Embryology, 2nd ed. Williams and Wilkins, Baltimore, 1969, p. 3.
15. Gordon, H: Genetical Social and Medical Aspects of Abortion. South African Med J, July 20, 1968, pp. 721-30.
16. Shettles, LB: Ovum Humanum. Hafner, NY, 1960, p. 60.
17. Davies, J: Human Developmental Anatomy. Ronald Press, NY, 1963, p. 3.
18. Dodds, GD: The Essential of Human Embryology, 2nd ed. Wiley, NY, 1964, p. 2.
19. Gilbert, MS: Biography of the Unborn. Williams and Wilkins, Baltimore, NY, 1938, pp. 2, 5.
20. Heisler, JC: A Textbook of Embryology for Students of Medicine, 2nd ed. WB Saunders, Philadelphia and London, 1901, p. 38.
21. Quimby, IN: Introduction to Medical Jurisprudence: Address Delivered by the Chairman of the Section of Medical Jurisprudence at the 38th Annual Meeting of the AMA, June 10, 1887. JAMA, 9:161-66, Aug. 6, 1887.
22. McMurrich, JM: The Development of the Human Body: A Manual of Human Embryology. P. Blakiston's Sons and Co., Philadelphia, 7th ed. 1923, p. 31.
23. Hamilton, WJ, et al: Human Embryology (Prenatal Development of Form and Function). Williams and Wilkins Co., Baltimore, 1945, p. 1.
24. Lejeune, J: The Nature of Man. In: Human Love and Human Life, JN Santamaria and JJ Billings, eds. The Polding Press, Melbourne, 1979.
25. Arey, LB: Developmental Anatomy, 6th ed., Chapters 2 and 6. WB Saunders Co., Philadelphia, 1954.
26. Ingleman-Sundberg, A, and Wirsen, C: A Child is Born: The Drama of Life Before Birth, photos by Lennart Nelsson. Dell Publishing Co., NY, 1965.
27. Patten, BM: Human Embryology, 3d ed., Chapter 7. McGraw-Hill Book Co., NY, 1968.

28. Rugh, R and Shettles, LB: From Conception to Birth: The Drama of Life's Beginnings. Harper and Row, NY, 1971.

29. Knaus, H: Fine Neve Methode Zur Bestimmung Des Ovulation Stermines. Zentrabl f Gynak, 53:2193, 1929.

30. Ogino, K: Ovulation Stermines and Konzeptionstermines. Zentrable f Gynak, 54:464, 1930.

31. Marshall, J: The infertile period: principles and practice. Helicon Press, Baltimore, 1967.

32. Hilgers, TW and Bailey, AJ: Natural Family Planning IV – The Identification of Postovulatory Infertility (in press).

33. Roetzer, J: The Symptothermal Method: Ten years of change. Linacre Quarterly, 45:358, 1978.

34. Vollman, R: Commentary at S-T Accreditation Seminar, St. John's University, Collegeville, MN, June, 1978.

35. Doring, GL: Detection of Ovulation by the Basal Body Temperature Method. In: Proceedings of a Research Conference on Natural Family Planning. The Human Life Foundation, 1972.

36. Marshall, J: Cervical-mucus and basal body temperature method of regulating births – Field Trial. Lancet.

37. Kippley, J and Kippley, S: The Art of Natural Family Planning, 2d ed. The Couple to Couple League International, 1979.

38. Billings, EL, Billings, JJ, Catarinich, M: The Atlas of the Ovulation Method, 3rd ed. Advocate Press, Melbourne, 1977.

39. Hilgers, TW: A Critical Evaluation of Effectiveness Studies in Natural Family Planning. Paper presented at the International Conference on Natural Family Planning, sponsored by the World Health Organization, October 8, 1979, Dublin, Ireland (proceedings are in press).

40. A prototype training program for Natural Family Planning Practitioners has been established at Creighton University School of Medicine. This program, the first such program affiliated with a school of medicine in the United States, is under the direction of Thomas W. Hilgers, MD. For more information, you may write to him at 601 N. 30th Street, Omaha, NE 68131.

41. Pope Paul VI: *Humanae Vitae* (On the Regulation of Birth). Encyclical Letter, July 25, 1968. U.S. Catholic Conference, Washington, D.C.

42. Taymor, ML: Infertility. Grune and Stratton, NY, 1978.

43. Steptoe, PC, and Edwards, RG: Birth after the reimplantation of a human embryo. Lancet 2:366, 1978.

44. Rock, J and Menkin, MF: *In vitro* fertilization and cleavage of human ovarian eggs. Science 100:105, 1944.

45. Hayashi, M: Fertilization *in vitro* using human ova. International Conference on Planned Parenthood 7:505, 1963.

46. Blandau, RJ: *In Vitro* Fertilization and Embryo Transfer. Fertil Steril (in press).

47. Edwards, RG, Bavister, BD, Steptoe, PC: Early stages of fertilization *in vitro* of human oocytes matured *in vitro*. Nature 221:632, 1969.

48. Bavister, BD, Edwards, RG, Steptoe, PC: Identification of the midpiece and tail of the spermatozoon during fertilization of human eggs *in vitro*. J Reprod Fertil 20:159, 1969.

49. Edwards, RG, Gonahue, RP, Baramki, TA, Jones, HW: Preliminary attempts to fertilize human oocytes matured *in vitro*. Am J Obstet Gynecol 96:192, 1966.

50. Edwards, RG, Steptoe, PC, Purdy, JM: Fertilization and cleavage *in vitro* of preovulatory human oocytes. Nature 227:1307, 1970.

51. Steptoe, PC, Edwards, RG: Reimplantation of a human embryo with subsequent tubal pregnancy. Lancet 1:880, 1976.

52. Bevis, DCA: Embryo transplants. Br Med J 3:238, 1974.

53. Hilgers, TW: The Intrauterine Device: Contraceptive or Abortifacient? Minn Med 57:493, 1974.

54. Mishell, DR: Assessing the Intrauterine Device. Fam Plann Persps 7:103, 1975.

55. Wheeler, RG, Buschbom, RL, and Marshall, RK: A Rational Basis for IUD Design and

Development. In: Intrauterine Devices: Development, evaluation and program implementation, Wheeler, RG, Duncan, GW and Speidel, JJ, eds. NY, Academic Press, 1975.

56. Landesman, R, Coutinho, EM, and Saxena, BB: Detection of Human Chorionic Gonadotrophin in blood of regularly bleeding women using copper intrauterine devices. Fertil Steril 27:1062, 1976.

57. Tatum, HJ: The New Contraceptive: Copper Bearing IUD's. Contemp OB/Gyn 1:61, 1973.

58. Gibor, Y, Zipper, J, Stewart, WC, et al: The Association Between the Amount of Copper on Copper-carrying IUD's and their Contraceptive Efficiency. J Reprod Med 11:209, 1973.

59. Jecht, EW and Bernstein, GS: The Influence of Copper on the Instility of Human Spermatozoa. Contraception 7:381, 1973.

60. Family Planning Perspectives. Study finds copper IUD inserted after coitus prevents pregnancy and provides continuing contraceptive protection. 7:151, 1975.

61. Connell, EB: The Uterine Therapeutic System: A New Approach to Female Contraception. Contemp OB/Gyn 6:49, 1975.

62. Martinez-Manautow, J and Aznar, R: Report to First International Planned Parenthood Federation South-East Asia and Oceania Regional Medical and Scientific Congress, Aug. 14-18, 1972. Sydney, Australia.

63. Contemporary OB/Gyn. Development of the Uterine Therapeutic System. 3:69, 1974.

64. Federal Register. Text of required patient information for IUD's. Intrauterine Contraceptive Devices: Professional and Patient Labelling. May 10, 1977.

65. Goldzieher, JM, de la Pena, A, Chenault, CB, and Wontersz, TB: Comparative studies of the ethynyl estrogens used in oral contraceptives – II. Antiovulatory Potency. Am J Obstet Gynec 122:619, 1975.

66. Physicians Desk Reference. 32nd ed., 1978, pp. 1646, 1538, 1532, 1817, 1257, 1222, 1825 and 967.

67. Physicians Desk Reference. 32nd ed., 1978, pp. 1646 and 1829.

68. Roe v. Wade, 314 F. Supp. 1217, Supreme Court No. 70-18, Jan. 22, 1973.

Reverencing
Human Life
In Its Generation

William E. May, Ph.D.

In an unforgettable homily given to a great crowd assembled for Mass on the Capitol Mall of Washington, D. C. on October 7, 1979, Pope John Paul II affirmed: "Nothing surpasses the greatness or dignity of a human person. Human life is not just an idea or an abstraction. Human life is the concrete reality of a being that lives, that acts, that grows and develops. . . . Human life is precious because it is the gift of God whose love is infinite; and when God gives life, it is forever."[1]

In proclaiming the surpassing preciousness of human life John Paul II was simply expressing the constant faith of the Church.[2] According to this faith a human being, the concrete bodily being endowed with human life, is a being of moral worth, a subject of inviolable and inalienable rights that are to be recognized by others and protected by the laws of civil society.[3]

Because human life is so precious, there is an obligation to reverence it not only in its being but also in its coming-into-being.[4]

The Church has always clearly taught the need for reverencing human life in its generation, and in his pastoral instructions to the American people Pope John Paul II eloquently summarized the principal elements of this teaching, particularly in his homily on the Mall. In that homily he in effect provided us with a practical agenda for reflecting on the subject, "Reverencing Human Life in Its Generation." For in it he spoke of the beauty of marriage, that indissoluble covenant of life and love wherein alone human life can rightly be generated and given the home it deserves for its proper development. In it he strongly condemned the terrible crime of destroying unborn human life, and he also alluded to the irresponsibility of contraceptive acts, which only two days before, in a talk to the bishops of the United States, he had clearly repudiated as seriously wrong when he emphatically ratified the teaching of the Church that had been reaffirmed by Paul VI in *Humanae Vitae.*[5]

Here I propose to show the truth of the following propositions: First, *human life can be rightly reverenced in its generation only when this life is begotten in an act that expresses the selfless and exclusive love of the spouses for each other;* second, *a proper reverence for human life excludes contraceptive acts and practices;* and third, *the deliberate intention to destroy unborn human life through abortion is an infamous crime that ought to be legally proscribed.*

Since others here will be concerned with the issue of abortion in detail, and since the question of contraception has already been treated from almost every perspective, I will devote greater attention to the first of the above propositions than to the others. Moreover, in discussing this proposition I will be concerned both with the general relationship between marriage and the generation of human life and with specific questions posed by the development of such technologies as artificial insemination and *in vitro* fertilization.

Reverencing Human Life and "Good Law"

Before taking up these propositions, however, there is a question of great practical importance that needs to be addressed, even if briefly, namely the relationship between a proper reverence for human life and "good law."

According to the faith of the Church so eloquently proclaimed by Pope John Paul II, human life is endowed with an inherent dignity and sanctity. As Paul Ramsey has noted recently, "The notion that an individual human life is absolutely unique, inviolable, irreplaceable, noninterchangeable, not substitutable, and not meldable with other lives is a notion that exists in our civilization because it is Christian." Professor Ramsey continued by saying, "and that idea is so fundamental in the edifice of Western law and morals that it cannot be removed without bringing the whole house down."[6]

The truth that every human being, the concrete bodily being endowed with human life, is a being of moral worth and the bearer of inviolable and inalienable rights is not, however, self-evident. This great truth is both a gift of divine faith *and* an achievement of human intelligence insofar as it *can* be made manifest to the human mind.[7]

Yet it is not a truth that all people recognize. Indeed, there is growing evidence that this notion of human life is losing its hold on the minds of contemporary men and women. At the beginning of the 1970's an editorial in *California Medicine* noted that "the reverence for each and every human life has . . . been a keystone of Western medicine. . . . This traditional ethic," the editorial continued,

> is still clearly dominant, but there is much to suggest that it is being eroded at the core and may eventually be abandoned. . . . It is not too early for our profession to examine this new ethic, recognize it for what it is, and prepare to apply it in a rational development for the fulfilment and betterment of mankind in what is almost certain to be a biologically oriented world society.[8]

As we begin the 1980's, there is perhaps reason to believe that this "new ethic" to which the editorial refers, the "quality of life" ethic, is becoming dominant in our culture and is being reflected in the mores and legal structures of our society.

The notions of the "sanctity of life" and of "the quality of life" are speculative in character, and it does not lie within the competence of civil government to determine which is true, nor can these notions be put into human minds by legislative action. I submit, however, that the *normative principles* associated with these two differing and contradictory[9] notions of human life are *not* speculative truths upon which reasonable persons may disagree, but are rather practical propositions or precepts that can be tested by what John Courtney Murray called the "exigencies of civil conversation."[10]

Among the normative proposals advocated by adherents to the quality of life ethic – and unfortunately we discover these proposals in the writings of several influential Roman Catholic theologians[11] – are the following: (1) Only those members of the human species who are

58

meaningfully and not merely biologically alive ought to be protected by laws against homicide;[12] and (2) in determining whether a proposed act or practice is morally justifiable one must assess its consequences and choose that act or practice that will bring about the greater or proportionate good, even if the act or practice is the sort or kind of act or practice that human agents cannot freely choose without deliberately intending to do evil, or without intending to violate the rights of other human beings.[13] Among the normative proposals associated with the sanctity of life ethic are the following: (1) Every living member of the human species, being equal to all other members of this species in its humanity, ought to be protected by laws against homicide; and (2) one ought not to choose freely to do evil for the sake of good to come.[14]

If these normative proposals are closely examined, one will discover, I submit, that those associated with the quality of life ethic conflict with more basic requirements of practical reasonableness, such as *good is to be done and pursued and evil is to be avoided,* and *one ought not to do unto others as one would not have them do unto oneself,*[15] whereas those associated with the sanctity of life ethic meet these basic requirements. In short, the basic moral principles or requirements of practical reasonableness[16] in terms of which the normative proposals listed can be tested for their truth or falsity are themselves self-evidently true, in the sense they can be recognized immediately by any reasonable agent as truthful requirements of purposeful activity and do not have to be shown to be true on the basis of anything prior to themselves.[17] These principles, and the norms that can be shown to be true in terms of them, constitute what Murray called "good law," inasmuch as they are "invested not with the sanctity that attaches to dogma but only with the rationality that attaches to law."[18] These principles are simply the human expression of what Vatican II called "the highest norm of human life," namely, "the divine law itself – eternal, objective, and universal, by which God orders, directs and governs the whole world and the ways of the human community according to a plan conceived in his wisdom and love."[19]

It is not possible to pursue this vitally important question farther here. My principal reason for introducing it is to combat any sense of political impotence that may threaten all who cling steadfastly to the beautiful truth that human life is indeed a precious gift of God and therefore endowed with surpassing dignity and sanctity. It would be wrong, and would violate the basic principles of natural reasonableness, to compel our fellow citizens to assent to the truth that human life is sacred. Yet human lives can be, and must be, protected in their being and in their coming-into-being even if this truth is not formally acknowledged. They can be so protected because the basic requirements of practical reasonableness, the "exigencies of civil conversation" upon which a just political order depends, can be shown to demand that free and morally upright citizens, no matter what their ideological differences, be willing to regard justice and due process of law as exigent for others, even those whom they merely recognize as fellow humans, as they are for themselves and those close to them.[20]

Marriage and the Generation of Human Life

In his homily on the Mall Pope John Paul II affirmed that human life is precious not only because it is a gift from a loving God but also because "it is the expression and the fruit of love." Continuing, he said, "This is why life should spring up within the setting of marriage."[21]

Practically everyone would agree with Pope John Paul on this. It is true, unfortunately, that many human lives do come to be in the wombs of mothers who are not married to the men who have impregnated them; but this is almost universally regarded as a tragedy, and rightly so.[22] It is a tragedy not because a new human life has come into being, but because this life, this being filled with human potential and "capable of love and of service to humanity,"[23] is beginning life in conditions that are unjust both to it and to its mother.

Today, however, some urge that responsible single persons (of either sex) or couples consenting to live together (whether of the opposite or the same sex) be recognized as having a right to give life to a new human being (either through heterosexual coition or through other generative procedures now available) so long as they are willing to give this life the care and education to which it is entitled. In addition, some urge that not every married couple has a right to have children, suggesting that marriage is not of itself a sufficient criterion for parenthood but that some further test be established and met before married persons can be considered to have a right to procreate.[24]

It is not possible here to address the questions these groups raise, although I believe that the evidence and arguments needed to respond to them will be substantively contained in the analysis that will subsequently be given of marriage, the marital act, and the generation of human life.

Of more immediate and pressing concern here are the views of those who believe that married couples may, if necessary, rightly make use of such technologies as artificial insemination and *in vitro* fertilization in order to generate new human life. I believe that a true understanding of marriage, of the marital act, and of the relationship between marriage and the generation of human life will show that such practices are morally irresponsible. Moreover, once this understanding is grasped, it should be clear that artificial insemination by a vendor[25] and *in vitro* fertilization ought to be legally proscribed.

1. The Meaning of Marriage: Marriage does not derive from faith in Jesus and membership in His body, the Church. Nonetheless the human reality of marriage, which is in truth a loving gift of God's creation,[26] is a reality inherently capable of being integrated into God's covenant of love and grace. In and through Christ it has indeed been so integrated for those who experience this reality "in the Lord," that is, as living members of His body the Church.[27] Thus it is legitimate to speak of a Christian understanding of marriage, one mediated to us through the faith and teaching of the Church. It is this understanding – one that can be commended to everyone – that I wish to articulate here.

The beautiful reality of marriage comes into being through an act "of irrevocable personal consent . . . whereby the spouses mutually bestow and accept each other."[28] This act, which alone can bring marriage into being,[29] is comparable to the irrevocable act whereby God has freely chosen us as the beings with whom He wills to share His life and love and to that irrevocable act whereby His only-begotten Son, become one with us in His humanity, has freely chosen to become indissolubly one with His bride, the Church. In and through this act a man and a woman give to themselves a new identity: he becomes *her* husband and she becomes *his* wife and together they become *spouses*. This act of mutual bestowal establishes the man and the woman as uniquely irreplaceable and non-substitutable spouses. "Not uniqueness establishes marriage, but marriage establishes uniqueness."[30] In the act that makes them husband and wife, a man and a woman promise conjugal or marital love to one another: in virtue of this act and of the marriage that it brings into being they have henceforward the right, the freedom, and the obligation to love each other with conjugal or marital love.[31]

Marital love is a unique form of human love, and what makes it to be unique is the fact that it is an exclusive kind of love. But the exclusive character of marital love needs to be understood rightly. Husband and wife are not, through conjugal love, locked in an *egoisme a deux,* one that cuts them off from other persons or excludes love of other persons.[32] Quite to the contrary, they are enabled, precisely in virtue of their marriage and conjugal love, one "merging the human with the divine,"[33] to realize "the goodness and loveableness of all people, in fact of all living things."[34] Nor is conjugal love exclusive in the sense the husband and wife are the "property" of each other. Such possessive language is utterly foreign to and destructive of marriage and of marital love.[35] Rather conjugal love is exclusive in that it is a love whereby the spouses give themselves to each other fully, committing themselves to a sharing of their whole life (a communion in being) and in that in and through it they are both made capable of and dynamically inclined to giving life and love to new human persons through acts of procreative marital love.[36]

2. The Meaning of the Marital Act: The exclusive character of marital love, the character that specifies it and distinguishes it from every other form of human friendship love, can thus perhaps be best understood by reflecting on the meaning of the act of which spouses, and spouses alone, are capable, namely the marital or conjugal act. Although the spouses may freely choose never to engage in this act,[37] and although this act is not necessarily the *greatest* expression of conjugal love,[38] it is certainly true that marriage is ordered to this act[39] and that it is the act in which exclusive marital love is "uniquely expressed and perfected."[40]

The marital act is the act of marital coition. This act exhibits, symbolizes, manifests the exclusive nature of marital love, and it does so because it is both a communion in being (conjugal love as unitive) and is the sort or kind of act in and through which the spouses are "open to the transmission of life" (conjugal love as procreative). This is the meaning objectively rooted in the marital act itself and intelligibly discernible in it; it is not a meaning arbitrarily imposed upon or given to the act.

The marital act is unitive, i.e., a communion in being or an intimate, exclusive sharing of personal life because through it and in it they come to know each other in a unique way, revealing themselves to each other. In and through it they become one flesh, that is, humanly and personally one, renewing the covenant they have made with each other in the act that made them to be spouses.[41] Moreover in this act husband and wife exhibit their complementarity as male and female; for this act is possible only because the male, who has a penis, is able personally to enter into the person of the female, and she is uniquely capable of receiving personally into her body, her person, the male; and her act of receiving in a giving sort of way is just as central to the meaning of this act as is the male's act of giving his person to her in a receiving sort of way.[42] The male cannot, in his act, give himself to the female, unite his person with hers (i.e., exercise the unitive power of his sexuality), unless she gives herself to him by receiving him, nor can she receive him in this self-giving way by the exercise of the unitive power of her sexuality unless he gives himself to her by letting himself be received by her.

The marital act is procreative insofar as it is the kind or sort of act – and the kind or sort of act *alone* – that makes it possible for husband and wife to exercise *maritally* their beautiful personal and sexual powers of procreation, of giving life to a new human person. It is, in short, the sort or kind of act that is "open to the transmission of life" in a marital and procreative way.

And finally, this act is *marital* because it is an act that *only* spouses can do. Unmarried persons may be able to engage in acts of sexual coition, but since they have not made themselves to be non-substitutable and irreplaceable spouses through the act of making them to be married persons, such acts are in no way the manifestation of an exclusive sort of love.[43] Moreover, this act is *marital* not only because married persons *alone* can do it, but also because it is the *only* sort or kind of act that married persons can do that other persons cannot do. Moreover, if married persons engage in sexual coition and in doing so choose either to repudiate its exclusively unitive nature by having disregard or even contempt for the feelings of each other or to repudiate its procreative character by making it to be the sort or kind of act *closed* to the transmission of life, they are not engaging in the marital act.[44]

Marriage, the Marital Act, and the Laboratory Generation of Human Life

Today it is possible to generate human life through acts other than those of heterosexual genital coition (whether this coition be marital or nonmarital). Artificial insemination has been practiced for several decades,[45] and more recently there have been some successful efforts to generate new human life *in vitro*, to implant this developing life within the womb of its mother, and to give this life birth.[46] Other noncoital and even asexual methods of generating human life have been proposed and may be capable of being used in the future.[47]

I believe that all of these methods of generating human life are irresponsible and that they violate the reverence due to human life in its generation. I hope to show that they are by first presenting a general argument and then by offering more specific and subsidiary arguments against artificial insemination by a vendor and *in vitro* fertilization.

The general argument can be formulated as follows. Any act of generating human life that is nonmarital is irresponsible and violates the reverence due to human life in its generation. But artificial insemination (whether by a vendor or by a husband), *in vitro* fertilization, and other kinds of laboratory generation of human life are nonmarital. Therefore these acts of generating human life are irresponsible and violate the reverence due to human life in its generation.

The minor premise of this argument does not need extensive discussion. Artificial insemination by a vendor is quite obviously nonmarital, and the same is obviously true of *in vitro* fertilization that would involve the use of ova and/or sperm from persons who are not married to each other. But artificial insemination by a husband and *in vitro* fertilization in which an ovum taken from the wife is fertilized by sperm provided by her husband are also nonmarital in nature, even though married persons or spouses have collaborated in the activity. Such procedures are nonmarital because they are *in principle* procedures that may be effected by persons who are not spouses, nor is the spousal character of husband and wife intrinsic to such procedures even when husband and wife collaborate in them. What makes husband and wife capable of participating in such activities is not their spousal union but the simple fact that they are beings who produce gametic cells, ova in the case of the woman and sperm in the case of the man.

The major premise, of course, requires argument for its truth to be made manifest. Here the first consideration, I believe, is that a human life, the concrete life of a being that is the subject of inviolable and inalienable rights, is not to be considered as a product inferior in nature and subordinate to its producers and subject to quality control. Rather a human life is concretely an irreplaceable being of moral worth. For a Christian, a human life is concretely a living word of God, a created word that His Uncreated Word became for love of us. Thus, like the Uncreated Word, the created word is to "be begotten, not made."[48] A marital act, which is as it were a word spoken by husband and wife in which they affirm that they are open both to sharing life and love with each other and to sharing life and love with a new human life, is as such an act that gives reverence to human life. In and through this sort or kind of act, then, a human life can be begotten. The *nonmarital* act of generating human life by fertilizing a woman's ovum with the sperm of a male or by further achievements of human technology does not speak this language. Such acts may "make" babies, and the babies made by them are indeed precious and irreplaceable human lives worthy of the same respect and reverence due to all other human lives, but they do not beget a child in and through an act of spousal love.[50]

A second consideration is that any act of generating human life that is in principle nonmarital in nature sunders the link between marriage, the love proper to marriage and exclusive to it, and the transmission of human life. But this is irresponsible. It is irresponsible because it is in essence a destruction of marriage itself. Marriage, exclusive marital love, and the procreation of new human life through the marital act are goods that go together. To attack one of these goods is to attack and do violence to the others. Our age sufficiently bears witness to the destruction done to the reality of marriage by denying the exclusive yet nonpossessive character of marital love[51] and by denying the goodness of spousal procreativity.[52] To deny the link between the marital act and the generation of human life is further to threaten the good of marriage itself and is thus irresponsible. But this is precisely what is done when the proposal to generate human life in acts that are by their nature nonmarital is made.[53]

In sum, the nonmarital generation of human life violates the reverence due to human life in its generation by making its generation an act of reproduction, thereby reducing human life to the level of a product subordinate to its producers; it further threatens the good of marriage itself and by so doing endangers human life in its generation inasmuch as one of the cardinal purposes of marriage is precisely to provide the proper structure for the responsible generation of human life.

1. Artificial Insemination: More specific objections can be brought against the generation of human life through artificial insemination. Artificial insemination by a vendor definitely violates marriage itself and the marital covenant, even if the husband should consent to his wife's being inseminated artificially by the sperm of the vendor. It violates marriage and the marital covenant because in and through the act bringing marriage into being the spouses have given exclusively to each other their whole persons, including their powers of generating life. In artificial insemination by a vendor the wife gives her power of generating life over to one who is not her spouse and in doing so violates the covenant she has freely made just as she or her spouse would violate this covenant by choosing to give over to another their sexual power of uniting intimately in coition.[54]

Artificial insemination by a vendor, furthermore, is an injustice to the child to be given life. This child has a right to know who his father truly is, and he has a right, from the father who has freely chosen to give him life, to love and care and help. A man who generates human life naturally and never even cares to know the children to whom he has given life or never shows love and care for them is rightly held in dishonor in society. Yet the sperm vendor is acting in the same way.[55]

Because artificial insemination by a vendor is so terribly destructive of marriage and is such a gross injustice to the children brought to life in this way, this practice ought to be proscribed by civil law inasmuch as a civilized society has the obligation to foster and protect the common good. And surely the common good demands that marriage be respected and honored within a society and that the right of children to the care and support of those who give them life be protected.

Artificial insemination by a husband does not, of course, pose as patent a threat to the good of marriage; and obviously the husband who seeks to have a child through the use of artificial insemination by his own sperm is willing to meet his parental responsibilities. For this reason I do not believe that it would be appropriate for civil law to prohibit this mode of artificial generation of human life. The practice, nonetheless, is morally irresponsible. It is irresponsible first because it commonly requires that the husband masturbate in order to provide the sperm needed for the insemination. Although many in our culture deem masturbation either morally neutral or positively good,[56] and although several Roman Catholic authors contend that masturbation for this good purpose (or other good purposes) can be morally justifiable,[57] the Church teaches, and rightly so, that masturbation is itself a gravely wrong action, the sort that a human person ought not freely choose to do.[58] To enter into this issue adequately here is not possible. I believe that the Church rightly teaches on this matter; the basic reason why the Church's teaching is true can be perhaps summed up as follows. To choose to masturbate is to choose to exercise one's genital sexuality in a nonmarital way, in isolation from a spouse. But this choice is immoral because in and through it we are acting in a way destructive of the goodness of our genital sexuality. The goodness of our genital sexuality consists in the power that it gives to us to become one flesh, in an intimate union of exclusive and life-giving love, with a person of the opposite sex to whom we have given ourselves, along with our genital sexuality, in an act establishing that person as the irreplaceable and non-substitutable one with whom we will share our life. Freely to choose to exercise our genital sexuality in separation from that person is thus to act against the good of genital sexuality.

Artificial insemination by a husband is also morally irresponsible insofar as it is in principle a nonmarital act of generating human life.

2. In Vitro Fertilization: The generation of human life by removing an ovum from a woman, fertilizing it extracorporeally with sperm taken from her husband or from another, and then implanting the developing human being into the womb of the mother in the hope that it will continue its development until viable outside the womb is immoral for several reasons in addition to its being a nonmarital mode of generation.

One of the principal arguments against the morality of this procedure is that it constitutes an unethical experimentation upon the child-to-be. The strongest form of this argument, as advanced by Paul Ramsey,[59] claims that *in vitro* fertilization can never be considered an ethical experimentation insofar as we can never come to know whether this procedure will irreparably damage the child-to-be without being willing to inflict irreparable damage. Some authors, among them Charles E. Curran,[60] LeRoy Walters,[61] and Albert Studdard[62] criticize Ramsey's position on the grounds that were it a sound argument it would likewise prohibit the generation of human life through heterosexual coition, inasmuch as one can never positively exclude the possibility of generating a child who will be irreparably harmed in its generation (through recessive genetic defects unknown to the parents or through mutations). Thus Curran and others claim that *in vitro* generation would be morally permissible if it posed no discernible risks to the child-to-be greater than those posed by heterosexual coition.

Even if we grant, for the sake of argument, that *in vitro* fertilization would not be an immoral type of experimentation were it known that it poses to the child-to-be no greater risks than heterosexual coition, it remains true that today *it has not been shown* that this is the case. For this judgment I rely on the testimony of qualified scientists, persons like Luigi Mastroianni, Marc Lappé, and Leon Kass.[63] Moreover, and perhaps this is the principal consideration behind Ramsey's argument, we can never come to know whether it does without experimenting in order to find out, and experimenting on the lives of the very children-to-be who are subject to risk. Since this entails a willingness to perform a nontherapeutic experiment carrying potential hazards to the subject on that subject without that subject's own personal consent, to do so is unethical.[64]

In vitro fertilization further raises the possibility that prior to implantation human lives[65] brought into being through the process will be "discarded" should an abnormality develop and that the human lives developing *in utero* will be killed through abortion should subsequent monitoring of their development disclose any abnormalities.

For these and other reasons[66] *in vitro* fertilization is an irresponsible mode of generating human life, one that violates the reverence due to human life in its generation. Moreover, the practice is advocated as a way of fulfilling the private desires, however worthy in themselves, of private persons.[67] Yet the means advocated to fulfill these desires, namely the practice itself, is one morally repugnant to many. To involve the government, which is to serve the common good of all the people, in such a practice is both an injustice and an infringement on the liberty of those who do not wish to see their government involved in promoting private interests by approving morally objectionable practices.[68] Therefore *in vitro* fertilization ought to be legally proscribed.

Contraception and Reverence for Human Life in Its Generation

Most people in the western world, including large numbers of Roman Catholics, believe that contraceptive intercourse[69] is a morally permissible way of controlling human conception. Their position, I believe, is well summarized by Robert Hoyt, who said: "Contraception doesn't seem to hurt anyone and it helps solve some serious problems; what could be wrong with it?"[70]

Since the morality of contraception has been extensively debated over the past decade or so, it is not my intent to pursue the issue at length here.[71] It may suffice, for our purposes, to reflect briefly on three aspects of the question: (a) the reasons for its widespread acceptance, (b) the basic reason why contraception is immoral, and (c) the relationship between contraception and reverence for human life in its generation.

It can be shown, I believe, that the practice of contraception is widely accepted in our culture because this culture is now contraceptive. By this I mean that persons growing up in Western civilization today uncritically come to accept what can rightly be called a "separatist" understanding of human sexuality. By this I mean an understanding that has severed the connection between the unitive and the procreative dimensions or meanings of human sexuality, deeming the former alone as the humanly, personally significant of sexuality and the latter as a mere biological function, subhuman and subpersonal in nature, completely subject to the dominion and control of human persons.[72] This separatist understanding permeates contemporary Western civilization. It is eloquently expressed by such molders of public opinion as Ashley Montagu and by many theologians. Examples will suffice to show this.

Ashley Montagu, for instance, stresses the need to distinguish sharply between sexual behavior and "reproductive" behavior. Sexual behavior is a way of expressing friendship with others and of experiencing pleasure. In past times fear of reproducing inhibited the expression of friendship and the experience of sexual delights, but now, with the technological ability to separate reproduction from sexual fulfillment, mankind is freed from this terrible fear.[73] Daniel Maguire emphasizes the need for us to take control of our lives and not let our lives be ruled by the merely biological rhythms of our bodies. One reason why we need to do that is we need to liberate personal sexual activity, wherein we can enter into an intimacy of love with another, from the tyranny of biological reproduction.[74]

Obviously persons who share this understanding of human sexuality find no problem whatsoever in accepting contraception. For them it is a marvelous gift of human intelligence, enabling persons to subdue nature and bring it under control. And this understanding, I submit, is pervasive in our culture. It is uncritically accepted as true. On close scrutiny, this understanding, however, reveals an understanding of the human person that is quite dualistic, one distinguishing sharply between the conscious, experiencing subject, and the body with its biological rhythms that this subject can use, now for one purpose, now for another.[75]

In contrast to this widespread understanding of sexuality and of the human person, the Church proclaims an understanding that sees a human person to be a living human body and understands human sexuality to be integrally unitive and procreative. In short, the Church holds that the power to give life to a new human being, the procreative dimension of human sexuality, is just as personal and just as human as is the power to share one's own life personally and intimately with another in sexual union, the unitive dimension of human sexuality. Thus the choice to reject either the unitive good or the procreative good of human sexuality is not morally responsible, inasmuch as this means that one is willing to do evil for the sake of some other good. This is precisely the point made by Pope Paul VI in *Humanae Vitae* when he said: "It is justly regarded that a conjugal act imposed upon one's partner without regard for his or her condition and lawful desires is not a true act of love, and therefore it goes against the requirements which the right moral order calls for in the relationship between husband and wife. By the same token, it must also be acknowledged that a mutual act of love, which jeopardizes the possibility of transmitting life . . . goes against both the divine design of marriage and the will of the first Author of human life."[76]

This judgment of Pope Paul VI, vigorously ratified by Pope John Paul II, and itself simply a re-affirmation of the perennial conviction of the Church,[77] is rooted in the belief that human fertility is a blessing, not a curse. It is good that human beings have the sexual power to give life to new human persons, and what makes it even more wondrously and providentially good is that this great good is indissolubly linked to that other great good of human sexuality, its ability to express the intimate, exclusive love of spouses for one another. To regard this great good as a non-good, simply because its continued flourishing would inhibit our participation in some other created good, is wrong, and it is wrong because it amounts to a falsification of reality and to a rejection of something that is truly a marvelously good gift from God. Yet this is precisely what contraceptive intercourse entails. Contraception entails this because what makes contraception to be contraception is the repudiation of the procreative dimension of human sexuality because *here and now* this dimension of our being is regarded as a non-good.[78]

Once we realize this we can see the relationship between contraception and reverence for human life in its generation. What makes our procreative sexuality so surpassingly good is that it is a personal power, given to us by God, enabling us to participate in His power to give life. It is a generative power, good in itself, and ordered to another good of the highest order, the life of a new human person. An attitude toward this power, deeming it a merely functional, instrumental value and of itself simply biological and subordinate to the one who can exercise it, can frequently give rise to an attitude regarding nascent human life as merely biological in nature and subordinate to the interests of "persons," that is, to the interests of those conscious and experiencing subjects who "possess" this great power. I believe that we have already witnessed the generation of this attitude. Many who defend contraception as a right of intelligent persons to control their lives by exercising dominion over reproductive functions likewise distinguish sharply between "persons," that is, bearers of protectable rights, and human beings. These persons, and among them we find such writers as Joseph Fletcher, Daniel Callahan, and Daniel Maguire, grant that a human life is generated when a human ovum is fertilized by a human sperm, but they regard this life as human only in a biological sense, perhaps "on its way to personhood," as Maguire puts it, but not as yet equal in dignity to the true persons, that is, conscious subjects, who have generated it.[79]

From this it can be seen that contraception is the gateway to abortion. When I say this I in no way mean to imply that everyone who resorts to contraception would resort to abortion. Yet it is indubitably true that many who do accept contraception do believe that abortion is morally justifiable, as a "backstop" to contraception and as "post-conceptive" birth control.[80]

Moreover, and this is very important, several widely used forms of "contraception" are, in fact, abortifacient in that they do not prevent conception from taking place but rather prevent the developing child from implanting within the uterus. This is the case of IUDs, and it is also true that the contraceptive pills now marketed in the United States are also abortifacient, at times, in their procedure. These pills seek to control birth, first by inhibiting ovulation. But should ovulation occur, they then seek to control birth by causing chemical changes in the mucus of the cervix to kill sperm. Finally, should sperm survive and fertilize the ovum, these pills "work" by preventing the developing embryo from implanting in the womb. Since users of these pills cannot know *how* they will "work," they manifest a willingness to accept abortion, provided that they know that the pills work in this way. At present most people are ignorant of this, but such ignorance is vincible.[81]

Because the use of nonabortifacient contraceptives, although immoral, is not a direct attack upon elements in the common good, civil law need not prohibit their use. But in my opinion, the terrible harms inflicted both upon women and embryonic human beings by IUDs and pills, justify governments to exercise their responsibilities to protect the life and health of persons within the community, and that therefore the legal proscription of abortifacient pills and IUDs is a matter for civil legislation.

Abortion: The Gravest Violation of the Reverence Due to Human Life in Its Generation

The Fathers of Vatican II, expressing the mind of the Church and at the same time articulating the deepest convictions of countless men and women, branded abortion as an "infamy," a crime comparable to genocide.[82]

I do not propose here to discuss this issue at any length, both because others at this workshop will address it at greater depth and because there is already such an abundant literature setting forth in masterly fashion the great moral and social evil of abortion.[83]

Abortion is the greatest violation of human life in its generation because it is the willful destruction of this life during a stage of its development when it is most defenseless and helpless. That abortion is the destruction of a human being with potential, not of a potential human being,[84] cannot reasonably or realistically be denied today in terms of what we know about the significance of conception.[85] And what makes a human being a being of moral worth is not any quality added on to that being's humanity, but its being a member of the human species.[86] Thus the choice deliberately to destroy this being is the choice deliberately and of set purpose to destroy the life of an innocent human being.

This sort of choice is not only morally wicked insofar as it violates such basic requirements of practical reasonableness that we are to do unto others as we would have others do unto us,[87] but also a socially irresponsible act. As Arthur Dyke once put it, the injunction "not to kill," "is part of a total effort to prevent the destruction of the human community. It is an absolute prohibition in the sense that no society can be indifferent about the taking of human life. Any act, *insofar as it is an act of taking a human life,* is wrong,"[88] and it is moreover an attack against the bonds holding human communities together.[89] But this is precisely what directly intended abortion is. For this reason it is not only morally abhorrent but an affront to the common good of society. As such it demands legal proscription. If some members of the human community are excluded on arbitrary grounds from the protection afforded by the law against homicide, then all members of that community are threatened.[90]

This paper began with a citation from Pope John Paul II's stirring homily on the Mall. It can conclude by making its own what he eloquently proclaimed toward the close of this homily:

> When the sacredness of life before birth is attacked, we will stand up and proclaim that no one ever has the authority to destroy unborn life. When a child is described as a burden or looked upon only as a means to satisfy an emotional need, we will stand up and insist that every child is a unique and unrepeatable gift of God, with the right to a loving and united family. When the institution of marriage is abandoned to human selfishness or reduced to a temporary, conditional arrangement that can easily be terminated, we will stand up and affirm the indissolubility of the marriage bond.
>
> When the value of the family is threatened because of social and economic pressures, we will stand up and reaffirm that the family is "necessary not only for the private good of every person, but also for the common good of every society, nation, and state" (General Audience, Jan. 3, 1979). . . . A distinguished American, Thomas Jefferson, once stated: "The care of human life and happiness and not their destruction is the just and only legitimate object of good government" (March 31, 1809).[91]

Notes

1. Pope John Paul II, "'Stand Up' for Human Life," *Origins: NC Documentary Series* 9.18 (October 18, 1979): 279.

2. See *Yes to Life*, edited by Daughters of St. Paul (Boston: Daughters of St. Paul, 1977). This is an excellent collection of source materials, from the *Didache* to the 1976 Pastoral Letter of the American Hierarchy, *To Live in Christ Jesus*, bringing together the consistent teaching of the Church on the reverence due to life and the sacredness of life.

3. See, for example, *Gaudium et Spes*, nn. 26 and 27.

4. I wish to note here that I am not claiming here that an *is* (the fact that a human being is a being of moral worth) of itself grounds an *ought* (the obligation to respect and reverence human life). The basis for our moral obligation to respect and reverence human life is the intelligent directive of practical reasonableness (i.e., a basic precept or norm of morality) that we are to do good and avoid evil and that life is itself a good *of persons*. On this see Thomas Aquinas, *Summa Theologiae,* 1a2ae, 94, 2.

5. Pope John Paul II, "An Address to the U. S. Bishops" (October 5, 1979), *Origins* 9.18 (October 18, 1979): 289.

6. Paul Ramsey, *Ethics at the Edges of Life: Medical and Legal Intersections* (New Haven: Yale University Press, 1978), p. xiv.

7. On the knowability of this, see Mortimer Adler, *The Difference of Man and the Difference It Makes* (New York: Meridian Books, 1968); William E. May, "What Makes a Human Being to Be a Being of Moral Worth?" *The Thomist* 40.3 (1976): 416-443.

8. *California Medicine*, "A New Ethic for Medicine and Society," September, 1970, 67-68.

9. These notions of human life are contradictory inasmuch as the one affirms what the other denies and vice versa. Since these notions are truly contradictory, and not merely contrary, one must be true and other must be false.

10. John Courtney Murray, S.J., *We Hold These Truths: Catholic Reflections on the American Proposition* (New York: Sheed and Ward, 1960), p.45.

11. Among Roman Catholic theologians who hold that not all members of the human species are subjects of protectable rights but that some, for instance fetal human beings, are merely biologically alive and "on their way to personhood" are Daniel Maguire and Daniel Callahan. For Maguire see *Death by Choice* (New York: Doubleday, 1974), pp. 199-202 (cf. pp. 7, 12-13) and also *The Moral Choice* (New York: Doubleday, 1978), p. 448. For Callahan see his *Abortion: Law, Choice, and Morality* (New York: Macmillan, 1970), along with the incisive critique of this work by Paul Ramsey, "Abortion: A Review Article," *The Thomist* 37.1 (1973).

Among Roman Catholics who accept the proposition that it is sometimes right deliberately and of set purpose to do evil so that good may come about are Josef Fuchs, Bruno Schüller, John Dedek, Louis Janssens, Charles E. Curran, Richard McCormick, Philip S. Keane, S. S., and Timothy E. O'Connell. For literature on this subject see McCormick's two essays in *Doing Evil to Achieve Good*, edited by Richard McCormick and Paul Ramsey (Chicago: Loyola University Press, 1979) and O'Connell's *Principles for a Catholic Morality* (New York: Seabury Press. 1978), Part III.

12. This proposition, which is latent in many if not most arguments to support abortion, the "benign neglect" of "defective" children, and mercy killing, is formally articulated by Michael Tooley, "Abortion and Infanticide," *Philosophy and Public Affairs* 2 (Fall, 1972): 37-65. For further discussion of this proposition, along with its analogs in contemporary literature, see William E. May, *Human Existence, Medicine, and Ethics: Reflections on Human Life* (Chicago: Franciscan Herald Press, 1977), pp. 93-105.

13. This proposal is simply a way of affirming that the end justifies the means. For the literature defending this proposition on the part of Roman Catholic theologians see the works of McCormick and O'Connell listed in note 11. This proposal has been devastatingly criticized by secular philosophers and religious ethicists. For the best criticisms, ones showing that this proposal simply cannot meet the requirements of practical reasonableness, see the following: Germain G. Grisez, "Against Consequentialism," *American Journal of Jurisprudence* 23 (1978): 21-72; Paul Ramsey, "Incommensurability and Indeterminancy in Moral Choice," in *Doing Evil to Achieve Good*, pp. 69-144; Alan Donagan, *The Theory of Morality* (Chicago: University of

Chicago Press, 1977), pp. 172-209. See also the essays by John Finnis and William E. May in *Principles of Catholic Moral Life*, edited by William E. May (Chicago: Franciscan Herald Press, 1980).

14. Christian writers, including Pope Paul VI in *Humanae Vitae*, have traditionally seen in Romans 3:8 the revealed source for the principle that we are not to do evil for the sake of good to come.

15. On basic precepts of practical reasonableness (the natural law, the law that is the participation within reasonable beings of God's eternal law; cf. *Summa Theologiae*, 1a2ae, 91, 2), see Germain G. Grisez, "The First Principle of Practical Reason: A Commentary on the *Summa Theologiae*, 1a2ae, 94, 2, *Natural Law Forum* 10 (1965): 168-196 (abridged in *Aquinas: A Collection of Critical Essays,* edited by Antony Kenny [New York: Doubleday Anchor, 1969], pp. 430-483); John Finnis, *Natural Law and Natural Rights* (Oxford: Oxford University Press, 1980), pp. 59-133.

16. The term "practical reasonableness" is used by Finnis, Grisez, and other contemporary writers in the same sense in which natural law has traditionally been used in moral thought.

17. On the self-evident character of the basic precepts of practical reasonableness see *Summa Theologiae*, 1a2ae, 94, 2. See also R. H. Armstrong, *The Primary and Secondary Precepts in Thomistic Natural Law Teaching* (The Hague: Martinus Nijhoff, 1965); Finnis, *Natural Law*, pp. 33-34.

18. See Murray, *We Hold These Truths*, pp. 45-50.

19. *Dignitatis Humanae*, n. 3.

20. On this subject, it is very instructive to consult the excellent study of Germain G. Grisez and Joseph M. Boyle, Jr., *Life and Death With Liberty and Justice: A Contribution to the Euthanasia Debate* (Notre Dame, Ind.: University of Notre Dame Press, 1979), in particular, pp. 24-58, 298-335.

21. Pope John Paul II, "'Stand Up' for Human Life," 279.

22. Unfortunately today many seek to avoid this tragedy by advocating contraceptives for nonmarried persons, with abortion as a backup. For a brilliant analysis of the failure of this policy see James M. Ford, M.D. and Michael Schwartz, "Birth Control for Teenagers: Diagram for Disaster," *Linacre Quarterly* 46.1 (February, 1979): 71-81.

23. Pope John Paul II, "'Stand Up' for Human Life," 279.

24. For proposals of this sort, see the work by the former Catholic priest, Robert Francoeur, *Utopian Motherhood* (New York: Harcourt, Brace and Jovanovich, 1972).

25. I use this term advisedly. In a recent article George J. Annas notes that the term "donor" is a misnomer and that those males who provide sperm for artificial insemination by women whom they do not even know should be termed "sperm vendors." Annas writes: "It is a contract in which the vendor is agreeing to do certain things for pay. . . . The continued use of the term 'donor' gives the impression that the sperm vendor is doing some service for the good of humanity." "Artificial Insemination: Beyond the Best Interests of the Donor," *Hastings Center Report* 9.4 (August, 1979): 14-15, 43.

26. On this see the excellent treatment of the Genesis accounts of creation in Edward Schillebeeckx, *Marriage: Human Reality and Saving Mystery* (New York: Sheed and Ward, 1965), ch. 1; see also Pierre Grelot, *Man and Wife in Scripture* (New York: Herder and Herder, 1965).

27. On this see again the superb discussion by Schillebeeckx of the New Testament teaching on marriage, in particular that of St. Paul in 1 Corinthians 7.

28. *Gaudium et Spes*, n. 48.

29. On this see the Council of Florence, DS 1327; *Casti Connubii*, par. 6. See the excellent discussion of the historical development of this teaching in Schillebeeckx.

30. Helmut Thielicke, *The Ethics of Sex* (New York: Harper and Row, 1963), p. 95.

31. The act of matrimonial consent is not an act concerning property rights. As Aquinas puts it, the act of matrimonial consent is precisely that, a consent to marriage and to all that marriage involves, and it involves a life of friendship between husband and wife, a friendship that is to be, next to the friendship between the individual and God, the most intimate of friendships (cf. *In IV Sent*. d. 26, 2, on matrimonial consent and *Summa Contra Gentiles*, 3, 123, on the greatness of conjugal friendship.)

32. On this see Josef Pieper, *About Love* (Chicago: Franciscan Herald Press, 1974), pp. 50-52; Dietrich von Hildebrand, *Man and Woman* (Chicago: Franciscan Herald Press, 1968); cf. also Erich Fromm, *The Art of Loving* (New York: Harper and Row, 1962), p. 55.

33. *Gaudium et Spes*, n. 49.

34. Pieper, *About Love*, p. 51.

35. On this subject it is instructive to consult what George Gilder has to say in his *Sexual Suicide* (New York: Quadrangle Books, 1973), ch. 2.

36. *Gaudium et Spes*, nn. 48, 50.

37. Man and woman become husband and wife in and through the act of matrimonial consent: the marital act does not make them to be husband and wife; it *is* marital *because* they are already husband and wife. They can freely choose not to engage in marital acts, and some Christians do make this choice.

38. It is important to emphasize this matter. I believe that the marital act is indeed an act that perfects and uniquely manifests married love, but it is by no means exhaustive of that love nor is it necessarily its greatest expression. There is a time for embracing, and there is a time not to embrace, and at times husband and wife can show greater love for each other by choosing not to embrace coitally than by choosing to do so.

39. On this see *Summa Theologiae*, 3a, Suppl. 48, 1.

40. *Gaudium et Spes*, n. 49.

41. On this see John Kippley, *Birth Control and the Marriage Covenant* (Collegeville, Minn.: The Liturgical Press; 1976), pp. 105-113; Dietrich von Hildebrand, *In Defense of Purity* (Chicago: Franciscan Herald Press), pp. 54-76; Mary Rosera Joyce, *Love Responds to Life* (Kenosha: Prow Press, 1970), pp. 8-26.

42. Here I wish to express my gratitude to Robert Joyce, who has developed beautifully the complementarity of male and female sexuality, describing male sexuality as "giving in a receiving sort of way" and female sexuality as "receiving in a giving sort of way." His presentation is given in *Human Sexual Ecology* (Washington: University Publications, 1980).

43. Here it is important to stress that what makes marriage is the irrevocable act of free consent establishing the uniqueness of the spouses for each other. When persons who have not made themselves spouses engage in coition, they cannot express marital love because they have not made each other irreplaceable, nonsubstitutable persons; each remains *in principle* replaceable and substitutable.

44. I seek to develop this idea further in "Conjugal Love," *The Catholic Theological Society of America: Proceedings of the Thirty-Third Annual Convention* (1978) (Bronx, N.Y.: CTSA, 1979), pp. 135-142.

45. A brief history of this practice is given by Gerald Leach, *The Biocrats* (Baltimore: Penguin, 1972), p. 82 ff.

46. Louise Brown, born in 1978, was the first child brought to birth through this process, and since then two other children have been said to have been brought to term whose lives began through *in vitro* fertilization. In the decade prior to their success with Louise Brown, Drs. Robert Edwards and Patrick Steptoe had made over 300 other attempts.

47. A good account of the different forms of laboratory reproduction and their combinations is given by Leach, *The Biocrats*, pp. 80-117.

48. These words are taken from the Nicene-Contantinople Creed.

49. Here it is instructive to cite Joseph Fletcher, "Ethical Aspects of Genetic Controls," *New England Journal of Medicine* (September 30, 1971): 5-6: "Man is a maker and a selector and a designer, and the more rationally conceived and deliberative anything is, the more human it is. Any attempt to set up an antimony between natural and biologic reproduction on the one hand, and artificial or designed reproduction on the other, is absurd. The real difference is between accidental or random reproduction and rationally willed or chosen reproduction. . . . It seems to me that laboratory reproduction is radically human compared to conception by ordinary heterosexual intercourse. It is willed, chosen, and controlled, and surely these are among the traits that distinguish *Homo sapiens* from others in the animal genus, from the primates down. Coital reproduction is, therefore, less human than laboratory reproduction – more fun, to be sure, but with our separation of baby making from love making, both become more human because they are matters of choice, not chance."

For a critique of this view see William E. May, "Ethics and Human Identity: The Challenge of the New Biology," *Horizons: Journal of the College Theology Society* 3 (1976): 17-36.

50. The position set forth by Pope Pius XII seems important to note here. He wrote: "A child is the fruit of conjugal union when this union is fully expressed by the bringing into play of the organic functions and the sensory emotions attached to them, and of the spiritual and disinterested love which animates this union. It is in the unity of this human act that the biological conditions of generation must be posited." "Address of His Holiness, Pope Pius XII, to the Second World Congress on Fertility and Sterility," in *Proceedings of the Second World Congress on Fertility and Sterility* (Naples, Italy, May 18-26, 1956) (Naples: Institute of Clinical Obstetrics and Gynecology, University of Naples, 1957-58): 1.40.

The view of Pius XII is reflected by Leon Kaas in "Making Babies – the New Biology and the 'Old' Morality," *Public Interest* 26 (Winter, 1972): 32-33 and by Paul Ramsey, "Moral and Religious Implications of Genetic Control," in his *Fabricated Man: The Ethics of Genetic Control* (New Haven: Yale University Press, 1970), pp. 50-57 and in his essay, "Shall We 'Reproduce'?" *Journal of the American Medical Association* 220.11 (June 12, 1972): 1480-1483.

51. Today many, by denying that spousal love is exclusive, advocate mate-swapping and "creative adultery." See Robert and Anna Francoeur, "The Technologies of Man-Made Sex," in *The Future of Sexual Relations,* edited by Robert and Anna Francoeur (Englewood Cliffs, N.J. 1973). Anthony Kosnik et al. imply that such unions might be morally justifiable in their *Human Sexuality: New Directions in American Catholic Thought* (New York: Paulist Press, 1977), pp. 148-149.

52. Here I am referring to the sequelae of the practice of contraception by married persons. I believe that it is not just an accident that a dramatic rise in the number of divorces has accompanied the widespread acceptance of contraception. One factor may be that this practice imposes heavy burdens on women, who are usually the ones most responsible for taking care to use spermicidal suppositories, jellies; wear diaphragms, take pills, etc. Serious studies need to be carried out on this issue.

53. Paul Ramsey notes the immediate and real threat that such proposals raise against the institution of marrige in his *On In Vitro Fertilization: An Educational Publication of Americans United for Life, Inc.,* Studies in Law and Medicine, No. 3 (Chicago: Americans United for Life, Inc., n.d.).

54. In *Fabricated Man,* p. 33, Ramsey observes that even those Christians who do accept contraception "do not separate the sphere or realm of their procreation, nor do they distinguish between the *person* with whom the procreation may be brought into exercise."

55. This was brought out quite clearly by Gerald Kelly, S.J., in his *Medico-Moral Problems* (St. Louis: Catholic Hospital Association, 1957), pp. 231-239.

56. Typical here is the attitude expressed by James L. McCary, *Human Sexuality: Second Brief Edition* (New York: Van Nostrand, 1979), pp. 106-107, where he holds that masturbation is simply a good way of coming to appreciate one's own sexuality. His work, incidentally, is widely used as a textbook in colleges, and is the required text for courses on human sexuality in the School of Nursing of The Catholic University of America.

57. Among those who hold that masturbation for artificial insemination by a husband is morally justifiable are Bernard Häring, John Dedek, Charles Curran, Anthony Kosnik et al. See, for example, Häring's *Medical Ethics* (South Bend, Ind.: Fides, 1972), p. 91 and Dedek's *Contemporary Medical Ethics* (New York: Sheed and Ward, 1975), pp. 92-102.

58. See *Persona Humana* (Vatican Declaration on Certain Questions Concerning Sexual Ethics, December 29, 1975), par. 9.

59. See Ramsey, works cited in notes 50 and 53 above.

60. Charles E. Curran, *Politics, Medicine, and Christian Ethics: Dialogue with Paul Ramsey* (Philadelphia: Fortress, 1973), pp. 210-219.

61. LeRoy Walters, "Human In Vitro Fertilization: A Review of the Ethical Literature," *Hastings Center Report* 9.4 (August, 1979): 23-43. Walters' survey article is most informative and comprehensive.

62. Albert Studdard, "The Morality of *In Vitro* Fertilization," *Human Life Review* 5.4 (Fall, 1979): 41-55. It should be noted that Studdard, while criticizing Ramsey's position as demanding too much, is nonetheless very much opposed to *in vitro* fertilization inasfar as it certainly entails at present an unethical experiment upon the child-to-be.

63. Luigi Mastroianni, in F. B. Gebhard, Schumacher et al., *"In Vitro* Fertilization of Human Ova and Blastocyst Transfer: An Invitational Symposium," *Journal of Reproductive Medicine* 11.200 (1973): 196-199; Leon Kass, "Babies by Means of *In Vitro* Fertilization: Unethical Experimentation on the Unborn?" *New England Journal of Medicine* 285 (1971): 1174-1179; Marc Lappe, "Risk-taking for the Unborn," *Journal of the American Medical Association* 286 (1972): 49.

64. On the ethics of human experimentation see my *Human Existence, Medicine and Ethics,* pp. 17-38.

65. Here I wish to stress that a human life is brought into being at conception. See literature cited in note 85, below.

66. Other reasons, among them the remote but real threat that this process will lead to programs of designing our descendants, are brought out by Ramsey in the essay noted in note 53.

67. The desire of married couples to have children of their own is itself a good and noble desire. The moral question has to do with the human acts that they may freely choose to fulfill this desire.

68. For a development of this argument, see Grisez and Boyle, *Life and Death With Liberty and Justice,* pp. 139-183. What they have to say about the involvement of government in voluntary euthanasia can be applied to this question of "private choice."

69. I use the term "contraceptive intercourse" to show that contraception entails the choice (a) to have coition and (b) to make this coition the sort of act that is closed to the transmission of human life. Many writers today, particularly Roman Catholics such as Häring, Kosnik, and others seek to confuse matters by referring to two kinds of contraception, natural and artificial. For a critique of their views see my "Contraception, Abstinence, and Responsible Parenthood," *Faith and Reason* 3.1 (1977): 34-52.

70. Robert Hoyt, ed., *The Birth Control Debate: Interim History from the Pages of the National Catholic Reporter* (Kansas City, Mo.: National Catholic Reporter, 1969), p. 11.

71. In my judgment the best literature showing both that contraception is immoral and that the arguments advanced, particularly by Roman Catholic writers, to seek its justification are wholly inadequate, are the following: Elizabeth Anscombe, *Chastity and Contraception* (London: Catholic Truth Society, 1977); Anscombe, "On *Humanae Vitae,*" in *Human Love and Human Life: Papers on Humanae Vitae and the Ovulation Method of Natural Family Planning from the International Conference, University of Melbourne, 1978,* edited by J. N. Santamaria and John J. Billings (Melbourne: Polding Press, 1979), pp. 121-127; Germain G. Grisez, *Contraception and the Natural Law* (Milwaukee: Bruce Publishing Company, 1964), chapters 3 and 4 (although written before many arguments by Catholics to justify contraception were developed, this book anticipates, in chapter 3, the basic moral principles by which these arguments were developed and criticizes them cogently); John F. Kippley, *Birth Control and the Marriage Covenant,* pp. 65-96; William E. May, "An Integrist Understanding of Human Sexuality," in Dennis Doherty, ed., *New Dimensions of Sexuality* (New York: Doubleday, 1979), pp. 95-124. See also my *Sex, Love, and Procreation* (Chicago: Franciscan Herald Press Synthesis Series, 1976).

72. Grisez brilliantly shows this in his "Dualism and the New Morality," in *Atti del Congresso Internazionale Tommaso d'Aquino nel suo Settimo Centenario,* vol. 5, *L'Agire Morale* (Napoli: Edizioni Domenicane Italiane, 1977), pp. 323-330. I seek to develop this point in "An Integrist Understanding."

73. Ashley Montagu, *Sex, Man and Culture* (New York: G. Putnam, 1969), pp. 11-14.

74. See Daniel Maguire, "The Freedom to Die," in *New Theology #10,* edited by Martin Marty and Dean Peerman (New York: Macmillan, 1973), pp. 188-189.

75. This is clearly reflected in the so-called "Majority Report" of the Papal Commission on the Regulation of Birth. For an analysis of this document see the works of Grisez and May noted above, note 72.

76. Pope Paul VI, *Humanae Vitae,* n. 14.

77. Germain Grisez and John Ford, S.J., have presented a cogent argument that this teaching of the Church has been infallibly proposed. See their article, "Contraception and the Infallibility of the Ordinary Magisterium," *Theological Studies* 39.2 (June, 1978): 258-312.

78. For a development of this, see my "An Integrist Understanding."

79. See the works of Maguire and Callahan cited above, note 11.

80. On this see Paul Marx, O.S.B., *The Death Peddlars* (Collegeville, Minn., 1971), pp. 4-9.

81. On this point see the pamphlet, *The Pill and the IUD: Abortifacient?*, published by The Human Life Center, Collegeville, Minn., 1978.

82. *Gaudium et Spes*, nn. 27, 51.

83. Among the best studies on this question are: *Abortion and Social Justice*, edited by Dennis Horan and Thomas J. Hilgers, M.D. (New York: Sheed and Ward, 1974); Germain G. Grisez, *Abortion: The Myths, the Realities, and the Arguments* (New York: Corpus, 1970); John T. Noonan, Jr., *A Private Choice: Abortion in the Seventies* (New York: Free Press, 1979).

84. For evidence and arguments to show that there is, in being, a human being with potential rather than a potential human being from the time of conception see Robert and Mary Joyce, *Let Me Be Born* (Chicago: Franciscan Herald Press, 1970); William E. May, "What Makes a Human Being to Be a Being of Moral Worth?"

85. The works cited in note 83 provide massive scientific evidence and reasoned arguments to show that human life begins with conception. Since several authors today, among them such Catholic authors as Charles E. Curran, argue that the phenomenon of twinning and the possibility of recombination definitely prove that there is not in being an individual member of the human species at conception it is important to note that good arguments have been advanced to show that twinning can be explained quite intelligently as a form of asexual generation of life, with the one twin giving rise to a sibling. On this see Benedict Ashley, O.P., "A Critique of the Theory of Delayed Hominization," in *An Ethical Evaluation of Fetal Experimentation: An Interdisciplinary Study*, edited by Donald G. McCarthy and Albert S. Moraczewski, O.P. (St. Louis: Pope John XXIII Medical-Moral Research and Education Center, 1976), pp. 113-134.

86. On this point, in addition to the works cited in note 7 above see Grisez and Boyle, *Life and Death With Liberty and Justice*, pp. 218-238.

87. Here the comments by Roger Wertheimer, "Philosophy on Abortion," in *Abortion: Pro and Con*, edited by Robert Perkins (Cambridge, Ma.: Schenkmann, 1975), are quite pertinent.

88. Arthur Dyck, "An Alternative to an Ethic of Euthanasia," in *To Live and to Die*, edited by Robert Williams (New York: Springer Verlag, 1973), pp. 101-102.

89. For a development of this, see William E. May, "Abortion and Social Identity," *The Jurist* 32 (1974).

90. On this whole question see Noonan, *A Private Choice*, and Grisez-Boyle, *Life and Death With Liberty and Justice*.

91. Pope John Paul II, "'Stand Up' for Human Life," 280.

Pro-Life
Evangelization

Reverend Benedict M. Ashley, O.P., Ph.D., S.T.M.

Rhetoric and Evangelization

My colleagues are dealing with the scientific and legal aspects of the pro-life struggle, and with its basic theological foundation. I will address myself to the problem of how we can evangelize our country so as to bring about a true *metanoia*, a change of mind and heart with regard to the rights of the unborn. Without this conversion not only will it be difficult to change our laws, but even if our laws are changed through political strategies, they will not be effective. Abortion was a wide-spread evil in our country before the Supreme Court decision, as it is today in Latin America where such laws still exist.[1]

A change of mind and heart requires both education and rhetoric. Abortion is a profoundly emotional issue, touching as it does the intimate aspects of sexual life. Consequently, a merely abstract, intellectual, educative approach is not sufficient; we must also touch the heart. Good rhetoric, however, is not an appeal to irrational emotion. It is an effort to bring intellect and emotion into harmony in a practical conviction. It must appeal to objective truth, but truth as it is found in a people's life experience. Evangelization is both education and rhetoric, it appeals both to heart and head, but it goes further and appeals to faith, to the working of the Holy Spirit in the depths of the human spirit to bring about a radical change of the way both reality is seen and decisions are made.

In this effort at evangelization we cannot presume universal good will. The abortion movement exhibits a truly demonic aspect, exposing the profound sinfulness of our society, its hidden hatred of its Creator. Some really evil people are involved, such as those who are making money out of abortion clinics, or who promote abortion to remove every barrier against irresponsible lust. However, we should assume, I believe, that the vast majority of people who support "free choice" as it is called, do so out of sincere moral conviction, and really do see the pro-life position as heartless or fanatical. Our problem of evangelization, therefore, is to try to understand the genuine values such persons of good will think they are defending, and to show that these values when consistently pursued lead not to free-choice but pro-life convictions.

To approach a problem rhetorically is to take our point of departure from an analysis of the audiences we are trying to reach and their particular concerns. Any individual belongs to one or more interest groups in our society. I believe we can identify six principal interest groups in America who tend to a free-choice view and whom we especially need to evangelize: (1) certain of our fellow Christians; (2) theologians and philosophers; (3) parents and families; (4) social activists; (5) physicians; (6) women.

I. Fellow Christians

Traditionally not only all Christians, but also Jews and Muslims, have opposed abortion as contrary to the will of the Creator. Certainly, today, Catholics are by no means alone in maintaining this tradition. Yet a great many of our Protestant brethren, including many active in the ecumenical movement, have parted company with us on this issue. Why?

Three factors seem to me especially important.[2] The first is that when Protestants seek to discover the will of God in their lives, they seek to be radically obedient to God, but they tend to consider it irreverent to inquire *why* God demands this or that. In other words, their ethical stance is essentially voluntaristic, not teleological. If they are theologically conservative they seek the answer to their question in the explicit commands of God found in Scripture. Some, therefore, conclude that "Thou shalt not kill" settles the question of abortion. Others point out that the Scriptures contain no explicit application of this command to the fetus, and hence reach the opposite conclusion.[3] If Protestants accept a more critical understanding of the Bible, they reject this "proof-text approach" and find the will of God expressed in the New Testament only in broad general principles of love and compassion. Consequently, they reject the Catholic effort to formulate detailed and absolute rules of conduct as a reversion to the Old Law contrary to the spirit of the Gospel. Thus, they are *prima facie* suspicious of the Catholic claim resting on church authority to impose a detailed rule admitting of no exceptions.[4]

A second factor is that to Protestants the Catholic conviction that human personhood begins at conception seems to rest not on biblical teaching but on merely philosophical grounds, which they do not regard as a secure guide for Christian living. It is not that Protestants deny that the fetus is a person. They simply see no way to settle such a question. Lacking any firm conviction on this question, they tend to believe that particular cases must be dealt with an attitude of Christian compassion on the basis of a balancing of the good and evil consequences. The basic Reformation understanding of the human condition is that each of us is *simul justus et peccator.* In a sinful world all our moral decisions are ambiguous and only the forgiveness of God can liberate us from the mixed character of our actions.[5] Hence, they view the Catholic effort to say that rejecting abortion is always right, and having an abortion is always wrong as only a way to justify ourselves, which will lead to the same judgment on us that the Pharisees incurred from the Lord. Therefore, while abortion is usually wrong, we dare not say it is always wrong.

A third factor is that many of the Protestant clergy today have found that what seems to help their people most in counseling is a psychotherapeutic approach which accepts the client where he or she "is," and then helps them resolve their moral dilemmas in a way they "can live with," assured of God's forgiveness.[6] Such an approach seems to help people grow in Christian responsibility without demanding they live according to idealistic norms which they cannot realize in their own lives, and which only lead to excessive guilt, depression, and rejection of religion. Consequently, the leadership in the development of abortion counseling centers was largely the work of compassionate Protestant clergymen, whose influence was a powerful one in the movement to liberalize anti-abortion laws.[7]

How then are we to find allies for pro-life among these Protestant friends? Clearly, it cannot be achieved by questioning their motives. Nor will we get very far arguing for the personhood of the fetus in its early stages, nor by proposing an absolute norm against all abortion. We must begin with what we agree on, namely, that almost all Protestants are just as convinced as we are that abortion is a tragic evil, the result of our sinful human condition, just as war or capital punishment. Hence Protestants are ready to agree with us that the recent great growth in the number of abortions is alarming, and that we need first to provide practical alternatives to abortion, and second to find ways to restrict the growth of abortion encouraged by various kinds of exploitation and secularist propaganda. This area of agreement is much greater than the area of disagreement, namely, concerning whether in true hardship cases abortion is always wrong. However, at present we are tending to give Protestants the impression that we do not want their cooperation unless on the basis of the support of an Amendment absolutely outlawing legal abortion.

Of course, from a Catholic point of view, the Protestant position seems open to the obvious objection that once abortion is permitted in hardship cases it will soon be more and more extended. Their answer is that this is true of every responsible moral position, hence we can never cease to turn to God in a constant moral vigilance, rather than to rely on laws. The conclusion, of course, is that morality can never become mechanical, but must always be prudential.

II. Theologians and Philosophers

Christian theology today is increasingly ecumenical and "foundational," that is, it attempts to address an audience which no longer has clearly defined denominational or credal positions. "Apologetics" is out of style, but in a sense all of theology tends to become apologetical, or hermeneutical since it attempts to find a bridge between the secular language of the contemporary world and the traditions of Christian faith.[8] In this effort the borderline between theology and philosophy becomes very vague, although theologians and philosophers live in different academic worlds. No wonder then that so marked a polarization is developing between the bishops of the

Church who are striving to support the mass of Christians in a traditional faith and the theologians who are more concerned to reach the increasing number of Christians who speak only a secular language as well as to open up the faith to non-Christians. This difference of orientation is bound to encourage serious tensions and painful confrontations.

In the matter of abortion this confrontation is evident at two points. First, some theologians question how the Church knows when personhood begins, since the Scriptures do not say, and Church tradition is not unanimous on the point. Has not the Congregation for the Faith in its "Declaration on Abortion" also admitted this?[9] Second, and more importantly, many theologians are questioning the notion of absolute moral norms. Their contention is not that morality is merely subjective, nor simply situational, but that it cannot be settled absolutely on the basis of the nature of the pre-moral object. Rather, they argue, in any concrete act the morality of the act is dependent on the intention, the circumstances, and the nature of the act – all three taken conjointly. This means that in theory, if not in practice, any moral norm that we might formulate in the abstract will admit of exceptions. I hasten to say that I strongly disagree with this theory of proportionalism, but I must admit that it has able defenders and it's widely influential in pastoral practice today both in the United States and Europe.[10]

Closely related to such theological positions, but developed by a different methodology, are the theories put forward by some philosophers to deal with the abortion problem. Modern philosophy whether of the analytic, phenomenological, or process type (the varieties with theological influence most evident on the American scene) is not convinced that the human mind can arrive at the natures of things considered as *noumena,* independently of what our minds read into them, since all these systems in one way or another assume the Kantian concept of truth as a conformity of things to the mind, rather than of the mind to things. Consequently, a person, in the strict sense, must be a self-conscious moral agent. I know that I am a person reflectively and I can be convinced that you are a person if I can communicate with you. But to say that a person exists with whom I cannot communicate, or to say that I was a person even before I became self-conscious is meaningless.

Hence a common solution given to the problem of whether the

fetus is a person is to claim that although the conceptus is, biologically speaking, a human being or member of the human species, it is not yet a person, but only at most potentially a person.[11] The human being becomes a person gradually by entering more and more directly into personal relations with true, adult persons and by becoming self-conscious and self-determining. To the objection that if this is the case, then infanticide would be no violation of the rights of a person, the answer is given that on the basis of socially agreed criteria society can impute human rights to the infant and to other human beings who do not fully merit such rights. Thus, these philosophers conclude that although the unborn child is not morally insignificant, its moral claims are inferior to those of the mother, and the more inferior the earlier its stage of development.

This line of argument has been reinforced by the attempts of some to revive the old Thomistic opinion of delayed animation (or "delayed hominization"). In a study published by the Pope John XXIII Center I have tried to show that granting St. Thomas' theological and philosophical principles, but using the more accurate biological data available today, this theory lacks any solid probability.[12] Aquinas, on the basis of the facts as he knew them, believed that until the end of the first or second month the embryo has no unified human structure, but was still undergoing formation by an agent *extrinsic* to it, namely a vital force or *spiritus* in the semen which remained some time in the mother's womb along with but distinct from the menstrual blood out of which it was forming the embryo. Thus, Aquinas thought it was contrary to the facts to suppose that at this stage the embryo was developing by an *intrinsic* vital principle, i.e., a human soul.

However, we now know that from the moment of perfect fertilization,[13] the embryo develops through a principle intrinsic to it, namely, the genetic code contained in the primordial nucleus, and later, through the "primary organizer" which appears in the blastocyst and then ultimately through the central nervous system. This genetic code embodied in this central organ in its various phases of development is not a mere "blueprint," but also (and this is the essential point) a vital capacity to develop the whole organism into a mature human being, and it is this capacity for organic self-development into what is phenotypically a human person that we call the human-life principle or human soul.

The only plausible argument that has been raised against this interpretation is drawn from the fact that sometimes in the earliest phase of development the embryo can split into twins. This is quite understandable, however, both biologically and philosophically, as a special case of asexual reproduction or cloning, without resorting to the far-fetched hypothesis that human ensoulment normally occurs only after the critical point when such splitting becomes impossible, a hypothesis which faces two great difficulties: (1) If before this time the embryo has no human soul (no intrinsic vital principle) what causes it to development to this point? (2) What agent produces the two human beings at this point, when the ovum and semen no longer exist?

None of these philosophical arguments are really new, and in recent years the pros and cons have been quite thoroughly explored in various publications, yet at present the discussion seems to have come to a stalemate. Why? It seems to me from a perusal of the literature that this polarization is due principally to two causes. First, the parties to the debate do not take each other very seriously, and for the most part fail to confront and answer the opposing arguments directly. Second, the hidden assumptions of both sides are seldom made explicit or critically examined. No wonder, since the personhood question cuts very deep!

To achieve a breakthrough in this debate, therefore, will require a prolonged dialogue between opposing views in an atmosphere which is cordial and respectful. Ordinarily we might assume that such an atmosphere would exist in the Catholic Theology Society of America and the Catholic Philosophical Association, and that having resolved our difficulties we would be in a strong position to create occasions for discussions on this topic with non-Catholics. However, the recent controversy over the CTSA task-force report *Human Sexuality* shows that this polarization exists to an embarrassing degree in our own camp.[14] Recent actions of the Sacred Congregation for the Faith will probably increase this polarization.

What could be done to create a more favorable atmosphere? I can only respectfully suggest that the bishops of the United States might serve a peacemaking and mediating role in this situation, by inviting interchanges in meetings or through joint publications by a wide spectrum of scholars under the chairmanship or editorship of persons committed to giving all parties an equal hearing and encouraging them to confront each other's arguments directly. An interesting model of this kind of high-level discussion is furnished by the magazine *Current Anthropology*[15] in which the editors first invite a scholar or scholarly team to produce a paper reviewing the literature on a current topic in the field and taking a thoroughly argued position on it. Then, before publication of this position paper, it is submitted to ten or twenty other specialists of the most varied tendencies to submit their criticisms. Finally, the paper and the criticisms are published together, thus giving a really fair view of all sides of the question as currently understood by experts. If we are to make headway on the theology of abortion and related questions concerning sexuality, some such even-handed forum is urgently needed. Let me say that, for my own part, I am convinced that the official positions of the Magisterium have little to fear from such debate. What is to be feared is when defenders and dissenters talk only to their own followers.

III. Families

Moving now from the level of theory to that of practice, we need to meet the concern of parents who realize that the majority of abortions now being performed are intended to save teen-age girls from premature responsibilities.[16] Some of these tragedies are compounded by the fact that the pregnancy is the result of incest.[17] These facts have been very influential in gaining support for the free-choice position, especially among Protestants who are otherwise opposed to abortion. Formerly, the situation of unwed mothers was very difficult because of public contempt and difficulty of finding a marriage partner. Fortunately, today public attitudes are much more compassionate. Nevertheless, a teen-ager is seldom ready to be a responsible mother, even if she wishes to keep the child, and her own education and maturation are seriously hampered. Thus many parents urge abortion on their daughters, and, even if the parents refuse consent, a Supreme Court decision guarantees the girl free choice.

Formerly, it was believed by many that the solution to this increase of teen-age pregnancies was sex education and the easier availability of contraceptives, but it is becoming ever clearer that not only does this not solve the problem, but contributes to it, by saying to the young that premarital sexual activity is normal in our culture. We can hardly expect teen-agers to take the pains to avoid the consequences of their acts, when we teach them in so many ways that society stands ready to help them avoid these consequences. Many girls believe that extramarital intercourse is excused when it is done spontaneously and therefore out of love, and that it is cheapened by the foresight and planning required for successful contraception.[18]

What is very difficult for our society to accept, is what the Church has said all along, namely, that young people need social control, the sanctions and supports of a sober style of life to help them use their sexuality in a truly human and responsible manner.[19] But I believe it is also very difficult for Church leaders in our country to accept the fact that they must engage in a long, unpopular battle not merely to attack the symptoms of this sickness, but to bring about a radical restructuring of the American lifestyle as regards sexual behavior. Matters have reached a point where individual parents are almost powerless to raise their children in a Christian pattern of life. The public media constantly present an image of sexual behavior incompatible with New Testament teachings, and this becomes embodied in school life, dress, recreation, and the whole milieu in which young people grow up. To fight this destructive image is to invite ridicule and automatically to "turn off" the youth and their parents whom we need to reach. Yet unless we work for a radical change in this lifestyle, we cannot succeed in greatly decreasing teen-age abortions.[20]

Why are we inclined to accept this new sexual ideology as if it were inevitable, a development to which we must simply passively adjust? We constantly hear predictions that in the future sexual freedom will certainly increase, and that this is the inescapable and desirable outcome of modern medical and psychological discoveries.[21] Such predictions rest only on the myth of ever accelerating economic productivity and unlimited technological control. Fortunately, at this moment the "crisis of limits" is beginning to expose this myth.[22] It is time then that the Catholic Church courageously propose a new model for American sexual life, a model rooted in the perennial Gospel and the natural law, yet taking fully into account all we now know from the life and social sciences. What the CTSA study *Human Sexuality* failed to do, has now to be done – to provide a program for action by Catholics to change American life radically in the interest of stable families.

IV. Social Activists

How puzzling it is that today so many who have been the most dedicated fighters for human rights for racial minorities, for women, for children, for the poor, for the abolition of capital punishment and of nuclear war, are now proponents of abortion, the denial of the rights of the powerless unborn! That paradox cries for an explanation. We also need to understand why so many people active in the pro-life movement seem indifferent to the other social teachings of the Church.[23] Recently I talked to a woman who was a vehement opponent of the re-election of Senator Clarke because he advocated both abortion free choice and the "give-away" of the Panama Canal! She was quick to cite the bishops' condemnation of abortion, but she seemed never to have heard of their advocacy of progressive social positions, which she regarded with a horror equal to her horror of abortion.

What is the underlying theological cause of these strange inconsistencies? In my opinion we Catholics do not clearly understand our relation as a church to American society or the ambiguity of the term "human rights" as it is used in public debates in this country. Most of us think of our country as essentially Christian, and our Constitution as founded on the Christian concept of natural law. While we perceive that Christian influence is waning, we attribute this to a process of "secularization" which we suppose is inevitable with the advance of modern technology. Thus we tend to think of *Roe v. Wade* and the growing gap between traditional Christian values and the American life as a betrayal of our former national ideals. Hence some Catholics identify with the right wing of the American ideology that urges us to return to our "old time religion" and our "old time politics."

However, a serious theological study of our national history will reveal that both the conservative and the liberal elites in our country are committed not to a Christian world-view and value system, but to Secular Humanism. Just as in communist countries today the elites are guided by the secular religion of Marxism born in the nineteenth century, so in our country the elites are guided by the secular religion of Humanism born in the eighteenth century under the name of the Enlightenment which molded the thinking of the fathers of our Constitution. We may admire our Constitution and respect its remarkable achievements, but we need to recognize that it is not a Christian document, but a Secular Humanist document which the Supreme Court has interpreted according to the theology of that same secular religion.[23]

This means that today we Christians are a minority religion in our country, just as are Christians in Poland or in Iran. Certainly we should be thankful that Secular Humanism is a more tolerant religion than is Marxism, but we should also recognize that this toleration has its subtler way of rendering our Church powerless. Our parochial school system has been pushed to the wall, our hospitals are more and more pressured, and we are being told that we have no right to impose our religious views on others by pro-life advocacy in the political arena.[24] The truth is that "human rights" mean different things to a Christian, a Marxist, and a Secular Humanist.

Once we have clearly recognized our real situation, we are in a much better position to speak and act according to our own convictions in relation to others whose quite different convictions we can respect, without being seduced. The fact that we are a minority in a country dominated by Secular Humanism does not mean that we are aliens, or disloyal, but it does mean that we are in friendly opposition, and that we must maintain a constant prophetic criticism of the dominant elites. As critics, however, we cannot commit ourselves to the ideologies of either the right or left wing in American politics, since both rest on the assumptions of Secular Humanism. Only by clearly recognizing this and saying it to our people can we achieve a consistent and united Christian stand. Pope John Paul II has begun to take leadership in showing how it is possible to agree with Marxism on some issues, and to criticize Secular Humanist society on these issues, while not committing ourselves to either side.

How then are we to approach the social activist groups in our country, whether of right or left, who are concerned with important social reforms? Our approach must be "ecumenical," if I may use that word in this connection. We must deepen our own commitment to the Gospel, while remaining open to finding areas of agreement and cooperation with others whose notion of "human rights" is fundamentally different from ours. In cooperating with conservatives who disapprove of abortion but advocate militarism, or with liberals who disapprove of militarism while advocating abortion, we must follow the classical principles of cooperation. Moreover, we must use a forceful and realistic political strategy which demands recognition and support for our legitimate interests in exchange for our support of the legitimate interests of others. We must no longer tolerate being used to give respectability to programs for social justice by groups who then ridicule us as fanatics when we advocate aid for parochial schools or pro-life. Thus while encouraging our Catholic people to become more conscious of their own identity, we should not withdraw into sectarianism and political isolation, but become more deeply engaged in the shaping of our nation's future.

V. Physicians

One of the most appealing arguments for abortion is, of course, the mother whose mental or physical health is a risk, or whose unborn child is suspected or known to be seriously defective. Anyone who has encountered the anguish of women trying to decide what to do in such situations knows that the argument for an abortion seems overpowering, particularly when we admit that the social support which a woman might reasonably expect to help her care for a defective child, or for her family if she should die or be incapacitated, may be very difficult to obtain. However, I must say that I think the main problem in such situations is the attitudes of the medical profession today.

The present education of physicians, even in medical schools under Catholic auspices, leads them to consider contraceptives or sterilization as the most practical way to prevent a difficult pregnancy; and if this fails, to consider abortion as medically proper.[25] Consequently, the woman finds herself strongly tempted to accept the physician's assessment. Of course most physicians today recognize that their obligation is to present the medical alternatives with their risks and benefits to the patient and leave the ethical decision to her. Nevertheless, their own ethical attitudes, which tend to be utilitarian, provide the context of the patient's decision and strongly influence its outcome.[26]

A growing danger here is with regard to the development of genetic diagnosis through the use of amniocentesis and other new techniques, and genetic counseling to assist parents who may beget seriously defective children or a mother who is actually carrying a defective child. While such diagnosis and counseling may have real benefits and in 90% of the cases reassure the mother that her child is normal, evidence shows that centers for such counseling commonly accept abortion as the routine way to prevent the birth of a child suspected or known to be seriously defective.[27] This problem is going to become more and more acute as more and more genetic defects are discovered, as laws requiring genetic screening of the population are proposed and as people discover that these techniques will tell them in advance whether the child is a boy or a girl.[28]

What can we say to physicians to enable them to see that abortion is never a "treatment" for any medical condition either in the mother or the child, and should be considered quite outside the limits of legitimate medical practice? In the past the Church has sponsored guilds for physicians and magazines like the *Linacre Quarterly* to help the individual physician remain faithful to Christian medical ethics in his personal practice. Today, however, medicine is an enormously complex "industry," in which professionals are highly specialized in their skills and are incorporated in large institutions, and these, including our Catholic facilities, are being fitted together in a national system.[29] The ethical standards of this complex are pluralistic, but are inevitably being drawn into the dominant ideology of Secular Humanism, which I have already described. Christians working in this system are constantly confronted with the problem of material cooperation with practices (by Christian standards) in themselves objectively evil, just as in the business, military, and political world.[30]

In the face of this situation the Church has got to develop a new approach to physicians and other health care professionals. Every diocese needs an ongoing program of continuing education for such professionals, not merely on "forbidden practices," but on the nature of the health-care profession and its obligations in the service of people. In particular Catholic hospitals need an active rethinking of their mission, their problems of cooperation, and whether they are providing such services as centers for instruction in Natural Family Planning, genetic counseling, and help to parents of defective children.[31]

VI. Women

We come at last to what at the present is the most difficult group to talk to about pro-life – women concerned about women's rights. Few women are really pro-abortion, but feminists are convinced that anti-abortion laws are radically unfair, and constitute a form of "forced labor."[32] Judith Jarvis Thomson in a well-known article has argued that a mother in having an abortion is not killing the child, but simply exercising her right not to host an unwanted guest.[33] Sometimes, this is absolutely against her will, as in the case of a rape victim.[34]

Sometimes it is against her will in the sense that she and the man have lost the gamble that a pregnancy will not occur, but only she has to pay the bill. Sometimes it is against her will in the sense that she could not have foreseen the state of her health or the defective condition of the child. Both justice and compassion, it is argued, demand that a woman not be forced to go through with a pregnancy against her will.

It is easy to refute the logic of these arguments, but the Church cannot meet them merely with logic nor with self-righteousness. How are we to convince women that alternatives to abortion are really practical for them? It seems to me that in the first place we have to admit that our record as advocates of the rights of women is flawed. I believe myself that, relatively speaking, the record of Christianity in this respect is the best of any religion, theistic or secular; but it is far from perfect. Our chief mistake, I believe, has been to appear to preach to women that motherhood is their vocation, and to stress its heavy obligations; when we have been far less clear and forceful in preaching to men that fatherhood is their vocation and its obligations are equal to those of the mother. Perhaps the real cause of the feminist revolt is the failure of men to be real fathers, whether in marriage, in public service, or in the Christian ministry.

Hence it seem to me that if we are to convince women that abortion is not their way to liberation, we have to be seen as very active advocates of their liberation, and at the same time advocates of fully responsible fatherhood. On most of the demands of the women's rights movement the popes have taken a positive stand, but the Church in the United States does not have the image of working actively to implement these positions.[35] Only as that image becomes clear, and feminists know that, in spite of our opposition to abortion, on most matters we will give them active and effective support, and that even as regards abortion we are making serious efforts to provide alternatives, I believe we will see a shift in their attitudes. We have only to recall how quickly the Samaritan woman changed her attitude, when she found that Jesus understood her problems and fully accepted her. In fact He gave her a ministry, different than that of His apostles, but of equal significance.[36]

Conclusion

Permit me now to summarize the approaches in addition to our work for better legislation, which I believe we should take to these diverse groups whom we are trying to evangelize pro-life:

1. With other Christians we need to cooperate to diminish the number of abortions through joint educational programs and joint efforts to provide alternatives.

2. With theologians and philosophers we should promote more occasions for overcoming polarization by a direct confrontation of positions in a cordial atmosphere, working again for a wider area of agreement rather than capitulation.

3. With families we should carry on a long term effort though a well researched social program and strategy to effect a radical revolution in the lifestyle of our youth, since nothing less will check the massive trend toward illegitimacy and abortion in this age group.

4. With social activists we must clarify the fact that Christians are a minority in this country with our own values which cannot be equated with those of either the right or left of the dominant elites. Consequently, we will cooperate on specific objectives with various groups, but will be captive to none. We consider pro-life one of our legitimate objectives.

5. With physicians and health care professionals we must work diocese by diocese for an ongoing program of re-education first of Catholic professionals to develop a consistent program of pro-life medicine.

6. With women we must make clear by vigorous action that we support most of the demands of the feminist movement, while refusing to cooperate with those few aims which we believe are really not in the interest of women. We must stress the equal responsibilities of men in family care.

Notes

1. Daniel Callahan, *Abortion: Law, Choice and Morality* (New York, 1970). MacMillan discusses the Latin American situtation, pp. 156-174. John T. Noonan, Jr., *Contraception: A History of its Treatment by the Catholic Theologians and Canonists* shows that even in the Middle Ages abortion was a common problem, pp. 200-213.

2. An excellent discussion will be found in James A. Gustafson, *Protestant and Roman Catholic Ethics; Prospects for Rapprochement* (Chicago: University of Chicago Press, 1978).

3. An anti-abortion stance from a Protestant view is well represented by Harold O. J. Brown, *Death Before Birth* (Nashville: Thomas Nelson, 1977). An argument from an evangelical point of view, based on the silence of the Bible, in favor of free choice can be found in C. E. Carling, Jr., "Abortion and Contraception in Scripture," *Christian Scholar's Review* 2 (Fall 1971): 42-48.

4. A summary with selected bibliography of the views of Protestant theologians can be found in James B. Nelson, "Protestant Perspectives," in *Encyclopedia of Bioethics,* edited by

Warren T. Reich (New York: The Free Press, 1978), 1:13-17. Nelson's own views can be found in *Human Medicine* (Minneapolis: Augsburg Publishing House, 1973), where he proposes the creation of a liturgical service to meet the pastoral needs of women who have made this difficult decision. "A pre- or post-abortion rite . . . could incorporate acts of confession, conscious acknowledgement that it is a human life which is being ended, and assurances of God's forgiveness. For any decision to abort involves an inescapable moral ambiguity, even when that decision in a given situation is the better and humanly most responsible thing to do" (p. 58).

5. A detailed discussion of the "ethics of compromise" from a Lutheran point of view can be found in Helmut Thielicke, *Theological Ethics* (Philadelphia: Frontier, 1966), pp. 482-577.

6. The current confusion between psychological and ethical counseling is well discussed in Don S. Browning, *The Moral Context of Pastoral Care* (Philadelphia: Westminster Press, 1976). The relation of these to spiritual direction is also dealt with in Benedict M. Ashley and Kevin D. O'Rourke, *Health Care Ethics* (St. Louis: Catholic Hospital Association, 1978), pp. 23-26 and 401-406.

7. For example, the recent book of Dr. Bernard Nathanson and R. N. Ostling, *Aborting America* (New York: Doubleday, 1979), in which a former proponent of free choice who was the director of an abortion clinic relates the experiences and scientific information which led him to a change of mind.

8. William J. Hill, O.P., "Unity and Pluralism in Contemporary Theological Developments," an unpublished paper given in the Continuing Colloquium, *The Church and Scholarship,* sponsored by the NCCB and The Joint Committee of Catholic Learned Societies and Scholars, October 18-20, 1979, analyzes this situation well.

9. Sacred Congregation for the Doctrine of the Faith, "Declaration on Abortion," *The Pope Speaks* 19 (1975):250-262, note 19. "This declaration expressly leaves aside the question of the moment when the spiritual soul is infused. There is not a unanimous tradition on this point and authors are yet in disagreement" (p. 256).

10. The key articles in which the theory of proportionalism is developed are now available in Charles E. Curran and Richard A. McCormick, S.J., *Readings in Moral Theology,* No. 1: "Moral Norms and Catholic Tradition" (New York: Paulist Press, 1979). A brief refutation with biographical references to other criticisms is in Ashley and O'Rourke, pp. 189-193.

11. A leading Catholic proponent of this philosophical position is H. Tristam Engelhardt, Jr., "The Ontology of Abortion," *Ethics* 84 (1973-74): 217-234, but it has been put forward in many forms; for example, Edward A. Langerak, "Abortion: Listening to the Middle," *Hastings Center Report* 9 (October 1979): 24-28.

12. Benedict Ashley, "A Critique of the Theory of Delayed Hominization," in Donald G. McCarthy and Albert S. Moraczewski, *An Ethical Evaluation of Fetal Experimentation* (St. Louis: Pope John Center, 1976), Appendix A, pp. 113-135. Most of the proponents of delayed hominization have largely ignored the biological data, but Gabriel Pastrana, O.P., "Personhood and the Beginning of Human Life," *The Thomist* 41 (1977):247-294, takes this data into account, argues from the same principles I do, and reaches the opposite conclusion. I believe, however,that when he contends that the first sign of ensoulment is the appearance of the "primary organizer" in the blastocyst, he overlooks the significance of the fact that the differentiation of this organizer in the blastocyst is produced by an even more primordial "primary organizer," i.e., the nucleus of the fertilized zygote containing the genetic code. If the appearance of the "primary organizer" indicates ensoulment, *a fortiori* so does the appearance of the nucleus of the fertilized zygote, and for the same reason, i.e., unified development requires a central organ, and the existence of a central organ, by Aristotelian and Thomistic principles, is evidence of ensoulment.

13. I say "perfect," i.e., normal, fertilization, because the fusion of the nuclear material provided by the ovum and sperm may be abnormal, with the result that the apparently fertilized ovum may fail to develop, or may develop only through a few phases and then be spontaneously aborted. Hence, it is not evident that such abnormal embryos (estimates of the percentage range from 15% to 69%) are really human beings at all. The ontological status of such imperfectly fertilized ova is quite different than that of a zygote which is normally fertilized but which suffers from a genetic defect. The former was never a human being, or even a true organism; the latter is a true human being but a defective one.

14. For a criticism of the seriously faulty methodology of this work see my review article, "From Humanae Vitae to Human Sexuality: New Directions?" *Hospital Progress*, July 1978, pp. 78-81.

15. *Current Anthropology*, edited by Cyril S. Belshaw, is published by the University of Chicago Press for the Wenner-Gren Foundation for Anthropological Research.

16. According to the *Catholic Almanac* (1978), p. 99, in New York State over half of the abortions performed are for young, white, unmarried women. In some states it is estimated that as high as 80% of the abortions are unmarried young women.

17. Incest is only a minor cause of illegitimate pregnancies, but it is a widespread problem. See George E. Maloof, "The Consequences of Incest: Giving and Taking Life," *ibid.*, 73-110. On its psychological dynamics see Karen C. Merselman, *Incest* (San Francisco: Jossey-Bass, 1978).

18. See John Ford and M. Schwartz, "Birth control for teen-agers: diagram for disaster," *Linacre Quarterly* 46 (Fall 1979): 71-81.

19. William T. Liu, "Abortion and the Social System," in Edward Manier, William Liu, and David Solomon, *Abortion: New Directions for Public Policy* (Notre Dame: University of Notre Dame Press, 1977), pp. 137-158, in a discussion of the world-wide situation concludes that the trend to easy abortion as an institutionalized feature of modern society is so strong that there is little chance that it will be reversed. Of course, what this means is that it, like war, cannot be reversed except by *radical* social changes.

20. Thus Robert T. Francoeur, *Eve's New Rib: Twenty Faces of Sex, Marriage and Family* (New York: Harcourt, Brace, Jovanovich, 1972), argues that modern medical technology has opened up twenty alternatives, all of which are apparently ethically acceptable, as to how we will live our sexual lives in the future. He even includes celibacy as one!

21. Daniel Callahan, *The Tyranny of Survival* (New York: Macmillan, 1973), surveys the basic ethical problems faced by a technological society.

22. Andrew M. Greeley, *The American Catholic* (New York: Basic Books, 1977), has shown that it is a myth that Roman Catholics in the United States constitute a right-wing, or conservative, bloc of social and political opinion. See also his *An Ugly Little Secret* (Kansas City: Sheed, Andrews and McMeel, 1977), pp. 37-46.

23. Cf. Ashley and O'Rourke, pp. 16-23. I use the term "Secular Humanism" for that worldview and value-system which developed in the eighteenth century (usually under the name "the Enlightenment") in conscious criticism and opposition to Christianity. It is agnostic as regards the existence of God or a future life, and places its hopes exclusively on the human power to solve human problems by the use of science and technology. It grants religious freedom to theistic religions as long as they remain of a private character, not entering into the political arena, but regards them as purely a matter of subjective opinion.

24. See the editorial on *McRae v. Califano*, "Do Catholics Have Constitutional Rights?" *Commonweal* 105 (December 1978): 771-73.

25. Ashley and O'Rourke, pp. 95-105.

26. *Ibid.*, pp. 77-80 and 199-200.

27. Jean Ashton, "Amniocentesis: Safe but Still Ambiguous," and Tabitha M. Powledge, "From Experimental Procedure to Accepted Practice," *Hastings Center Report* 6 (February 1976): 5-7, and Powledge, "Pre-Natal Diagnosis: New Techniques," *New Questions* 9 (June 1979): 16-17. A new method being developed may eliminate amniocentesis by using stray fetal cells in the mother's bloodstream.

28. Genetic counseling centers do not encourage abortion as a method of sex selection, but there is some evidence that mothers are having prenatal diagnoses for this purpose. Also, some genetic diseases are sex-linked, e.g. hemophilia.

29. Ashley and O'Rourke, Chapter 6, "Social Organization of Health Care," pp. 124-155.

30. *Ibid.*, pp. 197-199 and 283-86.

31. *Ibid.*, pp. 152-53.

32. Virginia Held, "Abortion and Rights to Life," in E. L. Bandman and B. Bandman, *Bioethics and Human Rights* (Boston: Little, Brown, 1978), p. 107.

33. Judith Jarvis Thomson, "The Right to Privacy," *Philosophy and Public Affairs* 4 (Summer 1975): 295-314.

34. Donald G. McCarthy, "Medication to Prevent Rape," *Linacre Quarterly* 44 (1977):

210-22. Also, Sandra K. Mahkor, "Pregnancy and Sexual Assault," in *The Psychological Aspects of Abortion,* edited by D. Mall and W. F. Watts (Chicago: University Publications of America, Sponsored by the Department of Obstetrics and Gynecology, Stritch School of Medicine, Loyola University, 1979), pp. 53-72.

35. Some excellent pastoral suggestions are contained in Ralph Raineri, "The Unwed Mother: A Parish Approach to the Abortion Problem," *Today's Parish* 10 (October 1978): 11-12.

36. I say "equal" not because I accept the view that an injustice is done to women by their traditional exclusion from ordination to priesthood (an exclusion which I believe rests on solid theological grounds as indicated by the declaration of the S. Congregation for the Doctrine of the Faith on this subject), but because I think that we need to give to the ministries of women a recognition and honor which makes it clear that they are not "second class." How this is to be done practically requires further study.

Is Abortion a Private Choice

John T. Noonan, Jr., Ph.D.

What I would like to talk about first is what Walter Jackson Bate, in his recent biography of Samuel Johnson, says was the characteristic gift of Samuel Johnson as a moralist. Johnson's strength, he says, was his ability to perceive "that rarest and most difficult thing for confused and frightened human nature– the obvious." That is what I should like to concentrate on in the first part of this presentation.

If you look back in history you can see splendid examples wherein people turn from the obvious to concentrate on something else. For me the most striking example is that of William Blackstone, who in his famous commentaries on the laws of England made the first attack on slavery that any legal writer had ever made. And having made that great attack in 1765, he so confined it that it applied only to England where there were at the most some 10,000 slaves, and it was totally inapplicable to the English colonies where there were actually millions of slaves. Now, that kind of displacement from the monstrous problem to the small problem, is, I think, only too characteristic of a moralist. It is not totally hypocrisy; it is somehow fear before the intractable nature of the huge problem. And in our present situation where the figures are monstrous, our moralists, and perhaps all of us, have *some* temptation to turn from the huge and shocking and obvious facts to wrestle with some small and more manageable problem. So I should like to address the obvious.

The Leadership Elite

The first obvious thing is that we are living in the first society in human history where an elite in the society supports abortion. Of course, there has always been abortion as there has always been murder and adultery. But no society that I know anything of has ever, through its leadership, supported abortion as a good. And that is the America in which we now live.

In this respect I perhaps differ a bit from the analysis that was offered by Father Benedict Ashley (see pages 80-94). I do not see ourselves (the anti-abortionists) so much as a minority but as a group that has been cut out of the leadership group. The majority might very well be with us.

If you look at the leadership, it comes in four principal components. The first, of course, is the media, which has in effect become the fourth branch of the government; which has become in effect a rival teaching church. The media can then be broken down into the leaders: *The New York Times, The Washington Post, Time, Newsweek,* and the three television networks. Those leaders are all solidly in the abortion camp, and, in their wake, virtually every metropolitan newspaper in the country is actively in the abortion camp.

I was reminded recently by the editor of the St. Louis *Globe-Democrat* that it was on our side, and I said that I would mention it. But that is the only newspaper that I know of any size, which is at all anti-abortion. And so, all of us, certainly those of us who are not immersed in these things all of the time, are brainwashed by a sea of pro-abortion news, which also blots out most anti-abortion activity. The media then is the first element of the elite.

The second is the Federal Judiciary, that group of several hundred men and women – mostly men, mostly upper-class, white males – who have created the abortion liberty as a constitutional right and who have zealously, beyond anything that could be found in preceding legal doctrine, promoted the abortion liberty. Justice Brennan in what was the immediate forerunner of the abortion cases,

Eisenstadt v. Baird, declared there could not be any restriction on the distribution of contraceptives to the unmarried, and did so asserting that there was no difference between the married and unmarried, striking at the very heart of both Jewish and Christian ethical tradition. Mr. Justice Blackmun in *Planned Parenthood v. Danforth,* decided in the bicentennial year, declared that the only way that he can imagine a parent or a spouse having a right to say anything about abortion is by delegation from the state. This is an approach which, of course, is a radical denial of the natural basis of the family, and which, of course, led to the conclusion that neither a parent nor a husband had anything to be legally recognized about abortion.

Well, the spirit of the judiciary is not confined to the Supreme Court. It permeates the Circuit Courts of Appeals and the District Courts. There is, I believe, only one federal judge whose opinion I have read which was very much against abortion. Within one month (January 1980) we have had the example in Brooklyn of a judge who arrogated to himself a power which the Constitution actually gives to Congress to appropriate money. Contrary to what Article I, Section 9, of the Constitution says, that only Congress can appropriate money, Judge Dooling has chosen to appropriate a very large sum of money to fund abortion. And in doing so, he has said woman is "very close to the right to be."

The third element of the elite are the great philanthropies – principally, the great philanthropies centered in New York City. These organizations have given both respectability and large sums of money to advance the abortion cause here and abroad. The fourth element are the doctors, particularly the doctors associated with the university teaching hospitals. The doctors have now as a group, with notable and heroic exceptions, swung over to the abortion side.

Now these four elements of the elite range from the liberal to the conservative. The actual philanthropists are usually very rich, the doctors are usually quite rich. The federal judges and the opinion makers come from the affluent strata of society and yet they cross the ideological lines dividing left and right, they cross party lines, and they make a powerful coalition. Not by, I think, conscious conspiracy, but by convergence they have come to be the abortion power. The country since 1973 has been in the grip of the abortion power.

Physiological Facts About Abortion

The second obvious topic I should like to address is the nature of an abortion. In the early stages of pregnancy it sometimes lightly referred to as a D and C, dilation and curettage. The term curettage refers to the use of a sharp knife on the being in the womb, a sharp knife which will dissect that being. If the pregnancy is somewhat more advanced into its middle stage, the preferred method is described as a saline solution. This injection of salt will have the effect of poisoning the being in the womb and bring about death by poison. At this stage, or even at a later stage, a third modern method of abortion is by prostaglandin, a powerful chemical compound which could be used to induce and facilitate labor to bring about a true birth. If it is used in powerful enough dosage it will instead have the effect of impairing the circulatory and respiratory systems, and again bringing about the death of the being by poison, or, alternatively, bringing about delivery at a stage where the being will be too premature to survive. Finally, there is hysterotomy, the actual delivery in no fundamental way different from a Caesarean delivery of a child, but in this case, delivery with the intention that the child will be too premature to live. There is also the use of a vacuum, which is one way that the knife is supplemented in the early stages: a Berkeley aspirator is used to vacuum the womb and dismember the being.

When you look at these methods, you are tempted to say that they are all methods of committing murder; and there is precedence among our separated brethren for such usage. Karl Barth in his book on *Church Dogmatics,* describing what he says was the great social evil of his day, uses the word "murder" to describe abortion. Dietrich Bonhoeffer, writing in the shadow of execution by the Nazis, also described abortion as "murder." Yet although there is this warrant in other theological traditions, it is not our theological tradition, and it is not common English or American usage. We have reserved the term "murder" for the killing of a being outside the womb. It inflames the dispute to use the term "murder"; but it does seem that one could use with perfect accuracy and justness, the term "killing." As to all of these methods in use, the knifing and vacuuming and poisoning, if you applied them to any other living thing, to a pig or a bear or a chicken or even a bug, you would say that you were *killing* that thing. Whatever the status of this object, you would have to say that these methods applied to the being in the womb are also methods of *killing.*

That brings me to the third obvious thing – the nature of the being in the womb. Now as to that, we are in the paradoxical position of having far more information than any previous generation and yet doing more damage to this being than any previous generation. Father Ashley, with admirable fairness and clarity, set out the arguments that have gone on among the moral theologians on ensoulment and hominization. I do not believe that any of them are at all relevant to the issues in the public forum or the issues that must be addressed if American society is going to be changed. The public facts, the indisputable and obvious facts, are, first of all, that we know now the number of chromosomes which are the human number of chromosomes. When those chromosomes are present, we have a human being and not a bear or a pig or a chicken. So from the very beginning we have the chromosomal count and we also have the sex determinant. So from the beginning we can say it's a boy or it's a girl, and no need to speak of an it. We also know now, and I speak of discoveries within the last twenty years, that the DNA-information molecule carries all the information which will determine the physical characteristics of that boy or girl. It will determine teeth and toes and nose and eyes and complexion. From the beginning in that DNA molecule the information is coded.

The great French geneticist, Jérome Lejeune, speaking in defense of life, compared this DNA molecule to a tape recording which contained all of the works of Mozart. Taking up that comparison, suppose someone had such a tape recording of all the work of Mozart; and there were no other scores or records of Mozart in existence. This single tape recording was all that was left. Then suppose that the person in possession of that tape recording found it inconvenient to have around his house and destroyed it, and when reproached, he said, "It was only potential. It was only potentially the works of Mozart. As long as I wasn't playing it, it was just another potential that didn't reach its actuality." Well, no one, I suppose, would accept that defense. Yet that is the defense so often heard for the destruction of this DNA - information molecule – that it is only potential. It is no more potential than that tape recording of Mozart would have been. It is as unique and as precious as any tape of the work of Mozart or any other human being.

We have also seen in the last twenty years a great development of the science of fetology, particularly pioneered by another defender of life, Sir William Liley in New Zealand. We know now that at 28 days there is a pumping heart. We know now that at 45 days there are EEG signs to be read of brain activity. CBS, a year and a half ago, even had on television pictures at about 40 days of the heart of the being in the womb, and at 70 days of a working brain. There can be no *possible* excuse to a generation given this information to believe that this brain and heart are the brain and heart of the mother. They are not the mother's body. They are a separate, and, demonstrably separate, human body.

We also know now that by about the hundredth day, at least, there are in place pain receptors and enough development of the central nervous system so that pain can be experienced by the being in the womb. I say that because we live in a country where in every state there are laws protecting animals from painful death. If a dog or a cat or even a cow is to be put to death there are criminal laws protecting that dog or cow or cat, who belongs to someone, from being put to death painfully. Yet, in our country, the being in the womb is without protection from death and without protection from painful death. Even now (1980) in Illinois a statute is being contested which will protect from pain; one can well imagine the Federal Judiciary striking that down as inimical to the liberty of the abortion-seeking woman.

I can put before you these facts of psychology and physiology and genetics, and, for some people, particularly people in our modern civilization, they will speak strongly. They will indicate the essential humanity of this being who is the object of an abortion. There are others who must be spoken to through literature. I believe here our leading writers have served us even in the course of writing accounts of modern life that in some ways accentuate the excessive liberty of modern life. Writers like John Updike in *Couples,* and Joan Didion in *Play It As It Lays,* have brought out the essential horror of taking the life of a child in the womb.

But perhaps no one has put the matter with greater clarity than someone one would least expect to have done it, a French writer who all of his life struggled with problems of belief/believer. André Gide wrote this in his diary at the end of his life as he looked back, having been present at the abortion by his sister-in-law:

> When morning came, "get rid of that," I said naively to the gardener's wife when she finally came to see how everything was. Could I have supposed that those formless fragments, to which I,

turning away in disgust was pointing, could I have supposed that in the eyes of the Church they already represented the sacred human being they were being readied to clothe? O mystery of incarnation! Imagine then my stupor when some hours later I saw "it" again. That thing which for me already had no name in any language, now cleaned, adorned, beribboned, laid in a little cradle, awaiting the ritual entombment. Fortunately no one had been aware of the sacrilege I had been about to commit; I had already committed it in thought when I had said get rid of "that." Yes, very happily that ill-considered order had been heard by no one. And, I remained a long time musing before "it." Before that little face with the crushed forehead on which they had carefully hidden the wound. Before this innocent flesh which I, if I had been alone, yielding to my first impulse, would have consigned to the manure heap along with the afterbirth and which religious attentions had just saved from the void. I told no one then of what I felt. Of what I tell here. Was I to think that for a few moments a soul had inhabited this body? It has its tomb in Couvreville in that cemetery to which I wish not to return. Half a century has passed. I cannot truthfully say that I recall in detail that little face. No. What I remember exactly is my surprise, my sudden emotion, when confronted by its extraordinary beauty.

I suppose if we all had the perceptions and gifts of Gide, we could convey to everyone considering an abortion the extraordinary beauty of the being they wish to destroy. It is part of the obvious before us.

Finally, in the list of the obvious I would put the number of abortions every year performed in the United States. Whatever the figures were before the Supreme Court decisions, and, of course, they were hidden in darkness and guessing, there has been an enormous increase. If you took the highest figures estimated, guessed at, by the pro-abortion side, there has been at least a 25% increase. And what we know now is that, supported by the elite, over 1,250,000 human beings are being legally killed each year in our country.

Suggested Pro-Life Actions

In the face of the obvious, what are we to do? Here I should like to turn to the area of positive action. In part, of course, our task, your task, must be education. We must educate as to these obvious things. We must pierce the barriers set up by the media. In particular we must pierce the linguistic disguises which have become fashionable. Even within our own camp, one hears the word "fetus" sometimes used to describe the child in the womb. Well, "fetus" is a term common to human and animal biology and tends to emphasize the common animalness, and it is not the word that was used in either law or common speech before. In law when you gave a gift in a will or a trust to unborn children you did not give a gift in trust to a fetus, you gave it in a trust to a child. That was the language of common experience. Still in our country, I suppose, you do not say to a woman, "How's your fetus?" A woman thinks of having a child or a baby within her, not a fetus. Common sense resists the efforts to bring the baby to the level of an animal.

Yet, the agencies of government use this term, and now the Department of Health, Education and Welfare has carried it one step further, with the creation of the term, "fetus *ex utero.*" That would seem to be a contradiction in terms; a fetus is a being within the womb and *ex utero* is, of course, outside the womb. What does HEW mean when in government regulations it speaks of fetus *ex utero?* It means a child who has been delivered in an abortion who is fated to die and who is an appropriate object for experimentation under the rules set by HEW. With this contradiction in terms, it has designated such an aborted baby.

A third, common term, particularly in medical circles, is "termination of pregnancy," as though ending the life of a human being were something like ending a cancer. It is a shameful covering-up of the truth. Because the hospitals and the doctors and the medical journals would be ashamed to have regulations and articles about the killing of children, they have provided this euphemism.

Finally, in this area of linguistic concealment, I suppose nothing equals the effort of Judge Clement Hanesworth. Two years ago (1978), dealing with a prosecution in South Carolina for murder of a doctor who had brought about the death by prostaglandin of a seven-month-old baby, Judge Hanesworth dismissed the case under *Roe v. Wade.* Then he went on to say that the Supreme Court has decided that "the fetus in the womb is not alive." Imagine the state of mind from which that can be put forward seriously. I suppose Judge Hanesworth would hesitate to say that people over 70 are not alive, or people under 10 are not alive, even if the Supreme Court should say so. He sees nothing particularly strange in solemnly making the grounds for his decision, that by legal fiat this being who is moving and kicking and has a beating heart, is still not alive for the purposes of the United States Constitution. Well, education to make the obvious plain, to pierce such linguistic disguises, is one great mission we can all engage in.

Secondly, there is a political mission. As to that, one can see in this country different levels of political response. I said I did not think we are a minority. In fact, the best opinion polls have always indicated that the great majority of Americans reject abortion on demand, reject abortion for nine months, reject the liberty as the Supreme Court has actually given it. They are often in favor of it as described in the press, but in fact are against what the reality is. In fact, the greatest center of opposition to abortion is among women. I do not believe we need to win over the majority of American women; it is already ours. Certainly there is an elite group that needs to be won over. But the great strength of the pro-life cause lies in the women of America.

With such strength in the grass roots, one sees it reflected in the political process. The state legislatures which are closest to the grass roots are most pro-life; then the House of Representatives has become solidly pro-life in its voting on abortion funding. The Senate, which is more immunized from popular pressures, is closely divided. The Executive Branch agencies are more immunized, and the Judiciary is the most immunized of all. I do not believe that the legal battle, the political battle can ever change everything. It is only one element of the culture. Yet we live in a country that is a legalistic country; law is an important element of the culture. We cannot abandon the legal and political fields. If we should do so, we would be giving up on something that is part, at least, of the mission of Christians, if not the mission of the Church.

Here I wanted to bring in as a kind of counter-reflection, the view expressed on politics in general by the great Pope for whom Pope John Center is named. In his *Journey of a Soul,* John XXIII wrote: "The sublime work, holy and divine, which the Pope must do for the whole Church, and which the Bishops must do each in his own diocese is to preach the gospel and guide men to their eternal salvation. And all must take care not to let any other earthly business prevent, or impede, or disturb this primary task. The impediment may most easily arise from human judgment in the political sphere, which are diverse and contradictory according to the various ways of thinking and feeling. The gospel is far above these opinions and parties." A serious question for you is how this sublime view of the preaching of the gospel relates to you in this great battle that is actually underway in the United States over abortion.

Questions to Be Asked About Abortion

Realizing that this is an answer you yourselves alone can give, may I say for myself that preaching the gospel is to give criteria, and to give light, and to provide ways in which parties will be judged and, above all, ways in which priorities will be drawn up. If you do preach the gospel you will provide the light in which persons will make their judgments on the taking of life in the womb. In particular, it seems to me that if the gospel is preached, Catholics and other Christians (because I believe that this is an ecumenical issue) will ask themselves, "Why are we against abortion in the first place?" The answer to that would seem to be, "because it is not within man's power to take innocent life."

Now if that is the reason for being against abortion it would seem that a question that the President must answer is, "Why am I unwilling to do anything to protect innocent life? If it would be wrong for me to take this life myself (as I suppose must be the premise of every one of those politicians who says he is personally opposed to abortion but will do nothing) how can I in conscience then provide the means by which abortions are carried out, either providing the facilities or the personnel or the money? How can I refrain from working to bring about some protection for these lives in the womb?"

I believe that one must respect the consciences of the politicians and the legislators and candidates who affirm that they are against abortion but will do nothing. Yet, at the same time, it seems a task for Christians, possibly for bishops, to say these consciences are wrong. They have misjudged. They have failed to make the *proper* moral evaluation and they are in fact directly cooperating in injustice in failing to protect innocent life, and they are even directly cooperating in killing when they provide the mean of taking innocent life.

A second question that Christians will certainly decide in the light of the gospel teaching you give them is the question of priorities. Now I know there is a great danger for the Church to seem to be putting its values in only one place or, as the code expression goes, "in becoming a single issue Church." But you know that that term "single issue

Church" or "single issue voting" is a slogan coined by the friends of abortion to embarrass the efforts made to rectify the situation. It has never been thought on any other political issue that you were wrong if you had priorities and made your first priority the basis of your voting.

I put to you three analogies, trying to bring out the difficulty that everyone faces of preserving all of the values and the necessity of choosing priorities. First, suppose a father wants to be present at the sports activities of his son and the music recitals of his daughter and yet has to earn a living. If sometimes he cannot go to those sport contests or attend the music recitals but says, "The first thing I need to do is to earn a living," is he to be said to be indifferent or callous about the cultural and sporting activities of his children, or is he to be said to have put first things first?

Or a second analogy. Suppose a parent has a child seriously ill in a hospital and a kind relative comes and says, "I would like to give your child a $3,000 scholarship to my college." If the parent says, "I'd rather you gave me the money to help with the hospital bills so that the child may live," is that parent to be called indifferent to education because he puts the health of the child first?

Or finally, a third analogy. Suppose a family's house is on fire, and one child is in danger within the house. And the firemen come and offer to save the precious books and memorabilia and photographs of the family. If the father says, "No, save the child," is that father indifferent to all the other values in the house? It seems to me that in each of those cases, for all of us, the priorities would be inescapable. As to which situation we are in, I would say for myself that we are in the situation of a burning house.

Now having said that much on education, I would like to say that I believe that none of this can be accomplished without the help of the Holy Spirit. I recently came across a passage by a great American writer who, a century ago, had the same faith in the Spirit. He was responding to a much smaller disaster — one on a micro-scale, the wreck of a ship, the *St. John,* which was bringing immigrants from Ireland to Massachusetts and was wrecked off the coast of Cohasset on the Grampus Rocks, with the death of 99 of the passengers and with the Captain and the crew rowing to safety in the only life boat. It would have been very easy to have been cynical and defeatist as the technocrats escaped to safety and the poor and helpless died. But that was not the response of Henry Thoreau who came down to Cohasset where the bodies had been washéd to shore and wrote these words on the scene. Thoreau said:

> Why care for these dead bodies? They really have no friends but the worms and fishes. Their owners were coming to the New World as Columbus and the Pilgrims did. They were within a mile of its shores. But before they could reach it they immigrated to a newer world than ever Columbus dreamed of, yet one of whose existence we believe that there is far more universal and convincing evidence, though it has not been discovered by science, than Columbus had of this. Not merely mariners' tales and some paltry driftwood and seaweed but a continual drift and instinct of all our shores. All their plans and hopes burst like a bubble! Infants by the score dashed on the rocks of the enraged Atlantic Ocean. No! No! If the *St. John* did not make her port here, she has been telegraphed there. The strongest wind cannot stagger a Spirit. It is a Spirit's breath. A just man's purpose cannot be split on any Grampus or material rock. But itself will split rock till it succeeds.

You will recognize the Psalm that Thoreau invokes, where God splits rock. With the help of that Spirit you must go on splitting rock until every nascent human being, every human life within a mile of the shores of birth, is safe.

Death Issues

Introduction to Death Issues

Vincent Collins, M.D., a Chicago anesthesiologist, has followed the development of life-prolonging technology since the famous allocution of Pope Pius XII in 1957 which affirmed the principle that one is morally obliged only to the use of ordinary means of prolonging life. Dr. Collins discusses in separate essays below the medical determination of death and the medical approaches to prolonging life and managing pain.

The lawyer who presents twin essays below on legal determination of death and legal efforts to provide "death with dignity," Dennis J. Horan, co-edited with David Mall in 1977 an impressive resource volume entitled *Death, Dying, and Euthanasia* (Washington, D.C.: University Publications of America).

Rev. Thomas J. O'Donnell, S.J., currently serving as a medical-moral specialist in the Diocese of Tulsa, contributed four essays below, one on the theological approach to the determination of death, and three short essays on three separate prolonging life questions. He has authored a textbook on medical ethics, *Medicine and Christian Morality* (Staten Island, NY: Alba House, 1976).

The introductory and concluding essays on the prolonging life issue come from Rev. Donald G. McCarthy, Director of Education of the Pope John Center and a priest of the Archdiocese of Cincinnati. In 1976 he edited a book on the prolonging life issue, *Responsible Stewardship of Human Life* (St. Louis: Catholic Hospital Association, 1976).

Throughout the ten essays which follow, one finds always the dynamism of developing medical technology facing the inevitability of eventual human death. Behind this basic confrontation one finds the inherent tension between prolonging dying and prolonging living. The next decade can only expect a heightening of that inherent tension.

Definition
of Death

Vincent J. Collins, M.D.

Our task is to define death and the dying process. Today in medicine we are faced with a major dilemma. It is the recognition of full, spontaneous, integrated living processes on the one hand, versus the recognition and determination of the failure of some of these functions and processes leading to what we would name as the state of death, or the diagnosis of death. The main question then is, "When do we declare death?"

In order to do this, we have recognized that traditionally two kinds of processes have been analyzed. These processes were and still are those of respiration and of circulation. Death has traditionally been defined as the absence of these two functions, but today we also must add to these two losses of function, the loss of function of the integrating controlling organ of our body, namely, the central nervous system.

Having said that, I would like first to identify the fact we have three kinds of death to consider when we look at the phenomenon of death as a whole. Number one is clinical death. This is actually the death that we are going to deal with and analyze in some detail here.

But we also recognize, secondly, biological death. This is a follow-up of the clinical death situation. It follows with organs which integrate together to form the whole of the body, that each one in its turn when required tends to fail and, in turn, we call this organ failure biological death if irreversible. The biological death may be of the liver, of the kidney, and, indeed, of the heart and circulatory system, and the failure of the brain as an individual organ; such organ failure and death is followed by biological death of the cells. And, thirdly, we have theological death, which is a subject for the theologians.

Now, turning to clinical death, we have to consider the fact that death is a diagnosis. The diagnosis is based on simple signs or symptoms or the lack of these signs and symptoms as we observe a patient who has a terminal illness or an acute insult. There is already in existence a deterioration of functions to the point where the functions are indeed all lost, but lost in a sequential manner for different organs. We recognize the sequence depending on vulnerability to insult and make a determination of whether or not we can reverse the deterioration of function or whether it is irreversible. This represents then, indeed, the fact that three kinds of adjectives must be applied. One is the absence of *spontaneous* function; two is the loss of the *integration* of function; and three is the loss of *reversibility* of dysfunction.

Now, we really can't deal with a full understanding of the dying process without really looking at what the components of living, of life itself, are. There is recognized among biologists and among clinicians the fact that there are just nine organ systems, each with specific functions, but what is most important with regard to these nine organ functions is the fact that they are all coordinated by the central nervous system and its other component, namely, the autonomic nervous system. In general, we will refer to both as the nervous system. The integration, the coordination, coordinates not only the function of respiration, it also coordinates the function of the heart and of the circulation and maintains and modulates this is so that a person can exist spontaneously, and is able to resist the threats of his environment and is able to cope with problems of stress.

I would point out that each of these organ systems has no capability of living without circulation. For example, we recognize that if the brain has lost its circulation and its oxygen needs for approximately five minutes, that not only will function of the brain cease, or deteriorate and then cease, but indeed, the structure of the various brain cells may be compromised and there will be a deterioriation or disintegration of the cellular structure.

However, I would like to add at this point that with the brain there is a four-minute capability to survive and with the heart an eight-minute capability – the brain without circulation for four minutes, the heart without circulation for eight minutes, will deteriorate functionally and then structurally. But, having said structure and function, I must point out that you cannot have function without structure. However, you can have a loss of function without the loss of structure and that is important, because it is on the basis of the loss of functions, not on the loss of structure, that we make the determination and the diagnosis of death. When spontaneous function is irreversibly lost, structure may not be destroyed, but death exists.

We view dying as a process. It progresses from diminished function to absence to permanent loss. The end point is called death. A state. We recognize first, that there is functional failure as we have already noted. At one point in time, if this is due to a natural process or disease or to an unnatural accident, then there may be a period of time in which we can reverse the deteriorating function and return it to a full, spontaneous capability. The organs can, in general, individually and collectively under the control of the central nervous system, be returned to a spontaneous capability and function. On the other hand, if a period of time has elapsed, and we have exceeded the vulnerability index, we come to a point where there is irreversibility of function and eventually, of course, there is structural change. When there is this loss of general regulation by the central nervous system specifically, as distinct from autoregulation of individual organs, if the brain has lost its capability to function, we can declare death. It is not necessary ever that one waits for structural change; only loss of function is the basic determinant of death.

I should like at this point to indicate that Pope Pius XII himself was an acute observer of life and of biology. On November 24, 1957, he himself enunciated to a group of anesthesiologists the following: "Human life continues for as long as its vital functions distinguished from the simple (biological) life of the organs, manifest themselves spontaneously or even with the help of artificial processes." But the task of determining the exact instant of death is that of a physician.

A fundamental question exists as to how a physician should act in the face of a catastrophe or terminal illness. There are three courses of action open to a physician. He may vigorously use all his technology and resources without regard to benefit of the whole person under all circumstances. Many times, using artificial methods merely prolongs the dying process. He may also, because of social and other considerations, perhaps from a misguided sense of mercy and because of urging on the part of the family, decide that he will actively terminate the life of the patient. This is euthanasia. It is a clearly defined concept. But deceptive modifications have been proposed and the term reaffirmed, namely, active euthanasia as against passive euthanasia. The first is a redundant term – euthanasia is recognized to be a deliberate act to end a life. Lastly, the physician can pursue a course of passive management of the patient.

The second term, passive euthanasia, is a contradiction – a deliberate act cannot be passive management of the patient who has developed an irreversible condition. The physician can withdraw ineffective techniques and procedures and allow the patient to die from his disease. What then is the alternative to euthanasia in terms of how we manage a patient? The alternative is "therapeutic rationalism." This means that, if a therapy or a measure is not effective and is not reversing an altered function or system to a spontaneous condition, then it should either be withdrawn or at the very beginning a decision should be made to withhold therapy that is evidently not going to be beneficial.

Now, what about brain death? We must recognize that the brain has several levels of activity. There is the highest level of activity in the cortex relating to thinking, to experiences, and to consciousness. There are subcortical levels of activity relating to reflex autonomic and emotional responses. There are mid-brain levels of activity concerned with special responses, cranial nerves and alertness, and there are pontile levels of activity modulating posture and respiration and, lastly, there is the fifth level, namely the medullary area, wherein the vital centers of respiration, circulation and cardiac action are considered to exist. In the loss of circulation, or the lack of oxygen, the vulnerability of the brain to such losses is usually manifested by an interruption of function of the highest centers. Unconsciousness occurs, coma develops, and then progressively the loss of reflex responses, both at the voluntary side. And, finally, the capability by the brain of controlling the function of other organs such as the kidneys and the liver, but more importantly, the respiration system and the heart, is lost. When this integration and control is lost by the brain and shows no capacity to return to spontaneous function, we, indeed, have a state that definitely can be called the death state.

There actually are ways in which we assess the various functions at the different levels of the brain. These are clinical criteria and test responses. We examine its ability to maintain spontaneous responsiveness. We look at the ability of the brain to maintain spontaneous respiration. We look at the ability of the brain to maintain a proper, adequate circulation. We look at the brain for its ability to control cardiac action. And when there is a loss of brain function control of all these other functions (the brain is a master controller) and when it is incapable of controlling, we now can state on a patient's chart, or the doctor at the home can make a statement, and declare that this patient is dead. It is not a difficult diagnosis. And the physician need simply state and declare that this patient is dead.

Death has always been determined by the absence of function – respiration and heart beat are functions. In today's technology, both can be temporarily suspended, but restored to full capacity. Likewise, brain function can be temporarily suspended, but restored to full capacity. Therefore, it is the irreversibility of these functions which determine death. Irreversible loss of brain function is paramount even as permanent loss of spontaneous respiratory or cardiac function.

Definitions of Death: Current Legal Status

Dennis J. Horan, J.D.

In the past nine years 25 state legislatures have passed statutes "defining death."[1] In addition, three state supreme courts and several trial courts have adopted brain death definitions.[2] This flurry of legal activity has been precipitated by much scholarly legal, medical and ethical writing addressing this topic which has been loosely described as definition of death legislation.[3] That description is somewhat imprecise since what really is at issue is not a definition of death but a decision as to whether an additional criterion for determining death may be made legal.

Obviously the issue is not an additional definition of death since what has been true remains true: you are dead when you are dead. One does not suddenly redefine the fact that a person is dead unless someone intends to define that as dead which is not dead. Such intended definitions have been part of the problem surrounding this issue as we shall discuss later.

Short Historical Background

Death is a diagnosis. Physicians have diagnosed death without the aid of statutes for ages. Why then in the last nine years has it become necessary for state legislatures and courts to embark on a sea of legislative controversy to do for the medical profession what it heretofore has been capable of doing for itself? Why, indeed, did the medical profession itself see a necessity for promoting legislative determination of brain death?

Part of the answer lies in the problems created by technology. As resuscitative technology became more and more sophisticated its use became more and more common. That use created a problem. People were maintained on machinery after a resuscitative crisis but they never regained consciousness. Physicians soon realized that that state of unconsciousness had become irreversible and that the brain was no longer functioning. The machinery was maintaining heart and pulse rate but was it maintaining the life of a person? A conceptual problem became obvious at this point.

In the past the diagnosis of death had always been based on the customary standards of medicine for making such a diagnosis: absence of circulatory and respiratory functions. Even the law accepted this standard although its inquiry into the problem had been practically nonexistent. In the current problem, however, circulatory and respiratory functions were present because a machine was causing them to be present. On what basis, then, could a person whose circulatory and respiratory functions were being maintained by machinery be declared dead?

A little common-sense reflection at this point would have solved the problem and headed off much of the unnecessary great debate which followed. Someone should have realized that circulatory and respiratory functions ceased when the brain ceased functioning and thereby caused the circulatory and respiratory systems to stop. In short, you were dead when your brain was dead.[5]

Instead, several movements began at this time among certain circles which caused even greater confusion. The brain is composed of several parts which include the medulla, cerebellum, midbrain and cerebrum. Cognitive function is thought to be a product of the cerebrum. One group of commentators proposed to society that once the cognitive function was lost then that person should no longer be considered a person and should be defined as dead. That is to say, death of the cerebrum alone, they argued, was the equivalent of death of the person.[6] In the brain-death debate this position presents the greatest danger to a value system which rejects euthanasia.

Two more groups of physicians added to the confusion. Fear of litigation made one group hesitant to arrive at the very common sense notion that you are dead when your brain is dead. Since circulation and respiration were being maintained, albeit artificially, they wondered if declaring such a person dead might lead to malpractice suits or criminal prosecution. This fear rendered them unable to act.[7]

Another group of physicians were interested in developing the medical art of transplanting organs from one person to another. In recent years organ transplantation had become possible and advances in technology were speeding its use. Organ transplantation, however, had to take place as soon as possible after death in order that the donor organs would be optimally viable in order to facilitate successful transplants. Delays in diagnosing death, it was said, make organ transplantation difficult if not impossible. This group of physicians saw brain death as a possible acceptable social means for curing what they considered an important problem stalling medical progress.[8]

A movement began to resolve the impasse. The medical profession was split on the issue but enough physicians feared the growing momentum of litigation to feel it necessary to seek legislative help in an area that should have been solved by the common-sense use of customary medical practice.

State Statutes

The impasse was broken by the passage of the first brain death statute in Kansas in 1970. Since that time 24 other states have passed similar statutes.[9] Basically what these statutes do or attempt to do is to retain the traditional standards for diagnosing death (absence of respiration and circulation) while adding another standard (brain death).

The statutes generally follow one of four different types.

The Kansas Model

One type is modeled after the *Kansas* law, which provides for alternative definitions of death – one based on brain death, the other based on absence of spontaneous respiratory and cardiac functions. The "brain death" alternative is as follows:

A person will be considered medically and legally dead if, in the opinion of a physician, based on ordinary standards of medical practice, there is the absence of spontaneous brain function; and if based on ordinary standards of medical practice, during reasonable attempts to either maintain or restore spontaneous circulatory or respiratory function in the absence of aforesaid brain function, it appears that further attempts at resuscitation or supportive maintenance will not succeed, death will have occurred at the time when these conditions first coincide. Death is to be pronounced before artificial means of supporting respiratory and circulatory function are terminated and before any vital organ is removed for purposes of transplantation.

Maryland, New Mexico and *Virginia* have enacted statutes virtually identical with the Kansas enactment, except that the Virginia statute requires the opinion of a consulting physician who is "a specialist in the field of neurology, neurosurgery, or electroencephalography" in addition to the opinion of the attending physician that there is an absence of spontaneous brain function. Commentators have criticized this alternative-definition approach on the basis that there are not two different ways of dying as the statute seems to imply.[10]

Absence of Brain Function

A second type of statute provides a determination of death based on absence of brain function, to be used only when the heart and lungs are artificially maintained. This approach is illustrated by the *Michigan* provision:

A person will be considered dead if in the announced opinion of a physician, based on ordinary standards of medical practice in the community, there is the irreversible cessation of spontaneous respiratory and circulatory function. If artificial means of support preclude a determination that these functions have ceased, a person will be considered dead if in the announced opinion of a physician, based on ordinary standards of medical practice in the community, there is the irreversible cessation of spontaneous brain function. Death will have occurred at the time when the relevant functions ceased.

Statutes in *Alaska, Hawaii, Iowa, Louisiana* and *West Virginia* are substantially similar except that the *Iowa* and *Hawaii* statutes require the opinion of a consulting physician as well as the attending physician.

American Bar Association Model

The *Tennessee* statute is an example of a third type of statute which follows the American Bar Association model and which reads:

> For all legal purposes, a human body, with irreversible cessation of total brain function, according to the usual and customary standards of medical practice, shall be considered dead.

This type differs in that there is no explicit provision made for determination of death based on respiratory and cardiac cessation although such is implied since brain death is a clinical diagnosis and it was not intended by the ABA that traditional means of determining death were to be susperseded by the statute. This approach is also followed in *California, Idaho, Illinois, Montana* and *Oklahoma.* California and Idaho require independent confirmation of death by a second physician.

Irreversible Cessation of Spontaneous Brain Function

A fourth type of statute provides that a person *may be* pronounced dead if he has suffered irreversible cessation of spontaneous brain function. Unlike the Tennessee statute this type of statute permits, but does not require, a physician to pronounce a person dead if brain function cessation has occurred. The *Georgia* statute is of this type, stating:

> A person may be pronounced dead if it is determined that the person has suffered an irreversible cessation of brain function. There shall be independent confirmation of the death by another physician.

Similarly, the *Oregon* statute provides:

> In addition to criteria customarily used by a person to determine death, when a physician licensed to practice medicine under ORS Chapter 677 acts to determine that a person is dead, he may make such a determination if irreversible cessation of spontaneous brain function exists.

A number of states make provision within their statutes for organ donation. The *California, Hawaii* and *Louisiana* statutes provide that a physician who makes a determination of brain death may not participate in the removal or transplantation of any organs of the deceased. Most ethical commentators see such a provision as necessary in order to remove potential conflicts of interest for the physician making the determination of brain death.[11]

Court Actions

Several courts have had the opportunity to deal with the brain death problem. Their basic approach has been to accept the testimony of the neurological experts on this issue. That testimony generally is provided so that instructions can be drafted which will indicate to the court and the jury an intelligible meaning and definition of brain death. In *Tucker v. Lower,* for example, which was one of the earliest cases to present the question of definition of death in the context of organ transplantation, the court instructed the jury that death occurs at a precise time, and that it is defined as the cessation of life; the ceasing to exist; a total stoppage of the circulation of the blood and a cessation of the animal and vital functions consequent thereto such as respiration and pulsation. This court initially refused to employ a medical concept of neurological or brain death in establishing a rule of law. In its charge to the jurors, however, the court did allow all possible causes of death to be considered by them including brain death. Unfortunately, the case was never appealed and there is no reported precedent. In addition the instructions are somewhat confusing.[12]

The Massachusetts Supreme Court accepted the concept of brain death in the case of *Commonwealth v. Golston.*[13] The court instructed the jury that brain death occurs "when in the opinion of a licensed physician based on ordinary and accepted standards of medical practice, there has been a total and irreversible cessation of spontaneous brain functions and further attempts at resuscitation or continuous support of maintenance would not be successful in restoring such functions." In *New York City Health and Hospitals Corporation v. Sulsona,*[14] a New York trial court in a declaratory judgment suit construed the definition of death in the context of the anatomical gift statute. The court held that the word "death" implies a definition consistent with generally accepted medical practice. Doctors are qualified to testify as to what the general standards are and a general standard of death based upon the diagnosis of brain death was found acceptable by the court.

Recently the Supreme Courts of Arizona and Colorado have accepted brain death. The Colorado opinion is illustrative.[15] A seventeen-month-old child was discovered to have breathing difficulty and was unresponsive. He was taken to a hospital where it was determined that he had been grossly abused and was not breathing. He was placed on a respirator. Subsequently the mother was arrested for child abuse and custody of the child was taken from her and placed with the Department of Social Services. The child's attending physician and consulting neurologist as well as the court-appointed neurologist testified that the child had suffered total brain death caused by extensive brain damage resulting from head trauma. The child had sustained multiple bruises, was completely comatose, was not breathing spontaneously and his respiration was maintained entirely by artificial means. He had no spontaneous muscular movements, no reflexes, including stretch or tendon reflexes and no response to even the most intense pain or other stimuli. Corneal reflexes were absent, his pupils were dilated and fixed, electroencephalograms were flat. The unanimous opinion of the physicians was that the respirator and any other artificial mechanisms supporting the vital functions of the child's body should be discontinued since the child had suffered brain death.

The court viewed the case as one involving the definition of death in Colorado. Conceivably, it said, the common law might be interpreted broadly enough to include permanent cessation of brain functions as one of the definitions of death since one of the common-law definitions of death was "cessation of life." The court rejected this definition as applicable to the circumstances here where respiration and circulation were being artificially maintained.

The court then proceeded to discuss modern scientific views, judicial decisions and comparatively recent legislation in other states as well as model legislation offered by the American Bar Association, the American Medical Association and the Uniform Commissioners. As the rule of this case the court adopted the provisions of the Uniform Brain Death Act which was created by the National Conference of Commissioners on Uniform State Laws.

The Colorado and Arizona cases illustrate our courts' willingness to act in instances where legislative activity has not provided a solution. Of significance is the Colorado Supreme Court's view that:

Under the circumstances of this case we are not only entitled to resolve the question, but have a duty to do so. To act otherwise would be to close our eyes to the scientific and medical advances made worldwide in the past two or three decades.[16]

Models Recommended by Professional Associations

The American Bar Association, The American Medical Association and the National Conference of Commissioners on Uniform State Laws have each adopted a recommended brain death statute. In each case the wording varies slight but the substance is the same. Each requires irreversible cessation of all brain function which can be determined in accordance with reasonable medical standards. The AMA version adds legal immunity for the physician.

The version adopted by the National Conference of Commissioners on Uniform State Laws reads:

> For legal and medical purposes, an individual with irreversible cessation of all functioning of the brain, including the brain stem, is dead. Determination of death under this act shall be made in accordance with reasonable medical standards.[17]

This definition is very similar to the definition adopted by the *American Bar Association* in 1975 which states as follows:

> For all legal purposes, a human body with irreversible cessation of total brain function, according to the usual and customary standards of medical practice, shall be considered dead.

The determination of death provision in the *American Medical Association* model bill states as follows:

> A physician, in the exercise of his professional judgment, may declare an individual dead in accordance with accepted medical standards. Such declaration may be based solely on an irreversible cessation of brain function.

Conclusion

Fortunately, it was early recognized that the use of cerebral to cortical death alone as an equivalent for brain death was unacceptable to medicine and society and constituted the introduction of euthanasia into our society.[18] Consequently, all of the brain-death statutes require total brain death or its equivalent as an acceptable standard. This standard is usually expressed as irreversible cessation of total brain function or equivalent language.

The brain-death statutes constitute a legislative determination which is really no different than the common-sense insight that should have been made by the physicians ten to fifteen years ago. When the brain has irreversibly ceased to function then the person is dead in spite of the fact that respiration and circulation are artificially maintained.

This is not to say that determining when the brain has irreversibly ceased to function is an easy diagnosis to make or that it is made easier by the existence of legislation supporting it.[19] What these statutes and cases are simply saying is that when your brain has irreversibly ceased all of its functions you are dead. When your total brain is dead you are dead. We should not confuse that acceptable medical fact by the also acceptable medical fact that in any given case it may be difficult to prove that the brain has irreversibly ceased all of its functions.

Irreversibility, of course, is the key. The diagnosis of brain death as irreversible is made with caution in the cases of children or drug-induced coma states. Experience has shown the difficulty of making the diagnosis in these instances.[20] That difficulty, however, is no greater than the difficulty medical practitioners experience in making many diagnoses and should not deter entry into the area of diagnosing brain death. The customary concern and caution of physicians, including even transplant physicians, will deter hasty diagnoses and will protect patients. The history of the slow development of brain death and its cautious use by the medical profession are proof of the profession's concern for the well-being of the patient, even dying patients.

Another key is the universally accepted criterion that brain death must be total. All brain centers must be dead. Death of the cortex alone has been correctly rejected by state legislatures and ethical commentators as the introduction of euthanasia which is contrary to our law. Karen Quinlan is in deep coma; she is not dead.

Some have argued that brain death is an acceptable criterion for death only if the words "brain death" are merely other words for saying the complete destruction of the entire brain.[21] If by destruction is meant the irreversible cessation of all neuronal activity, then understanding the issue in that fashion presents no insurmountable problems.[22]

A more significant problem in my judgment is what direction the law would take in the absence of the currently existing statutes.

All of the currently existing statutes require total brain death. Thus, the fear of introduction of euthanasia through brain death is, as I have argued elsewhere, obviated.[23] Without such legislation the avenue is left open for courts through judicial pronouncement to accept other but lesser standards of brain death if supported by competent neurological testimony. If that testimony supports only cerebral brain death as death, only a judge very sophisticated in these medico-legal problems would understand and be able to overcome the thrust of such ideologically oriented expert testimony.

The important problem is that without brain-death legislation requiring total brain death courts may unwittingly accept a much lesser standard and create even greater problems for society. Thus, legislation limiting the concept of brain death to the total destruction of the brain is beneficial and does not undermine any of the values we seek to support. Indeed, total-brain-death legislation enhances those values by prohibiting euthanasia and allowing only those to be declared dead who are really dead.

Notes

1. Ala. Act. 165, 1979; Alaska Stat. S.09.65.120; Ark. Stat. Ann. S.82-537; Cal. Health & Safety Code S.7180; Conn. Public Act 79-556; Ga. Code & 88-1715.1; Haw. Rev. Stat. S.327 C-1; Idaho Code S.54-1819; Ill. Rev. Stat. Ch. 110 1/2, S.302; Iowa Code S.702.8; Kan. Stat. S.77-202; La. Civ. Code Ann. art. 9:111; Md. Ann. Code art. 43, S.54F; Mich. Comp. Laws S.14.228 (2); Mont. Rev. Codes Ann. S.50-22-101; Nev. Stats. Ch. 451 (S.B. No. 5, ch. 162, Sixtieth Sess., 1979); N.M. Stat. Ann. S.1-2-2; N.C. Gen. Stat. S.90-322; Okla. Stat. tit. 63 S.1-301; Or. Rev. Stat. S.146.087; Tenn. Code Ann. 53-459; 1979 Tex. Sess. Law Serv., p. 368; Va. Code S.54-325.7; W. Va. Code S.16-19-1; and Wyo. Stat. S.35-19-101.

2. *Lovato et al. v. District Court et al.,* Supreme Court of Colorado, No. 79 SA 407 dec. 10-15-79; *Commonwealth v. Golston,* 373 Mass. 249, 366 N.E. 2d 744 (1977) cert. den. 434 U.S. 1039, 98 S.Ct. 777, 54 L.Ed. 2d 788 (1978) (Court adopts brain death as alternative definition of death).

See also: *State v. Shaffer,* 223 Kan. 244, 574 P. 2d 205 (1977) (upholding constitutionality of Kansas brain death statute); *Cranmore v. State,* 85 Wis. 2d 722, 271 N.W. 2d 402 (1978) (error not to instruct jury on what constitutes death); *State v. Brown,* 8 Oreg. App. 72 (1971) (gunshot wound rather than termination of life supports was cause of death); *Tucker v. Lower,* No. 2381 Richmond, Virginia, L. & Eq. Ct., May 23, 1972 (jury instructed that it can consider brain death as an alternative definition of death); *People v. Lyons,* 15 Criminal Law Reporter 2240, Ca. Super. Ct. (1974) (court instructed jury that victim legally dead from gunshot wound because of brain death before respirator turned off); *New York City Health and Hospitals Corp. v. Sulsona,* 367 N.Y.S. 2d 686 (1975) (court declares brain death as an alternative definition of death).

3. See e.g.: Horan, D.J., *Euthanasia and Brain Death: Ethical and Legal Considerations,* 315 Annals of the New York Academy of Sciences 363-375, Nov. 17, 1978 (this entire volume is devoted to the issue of brain death); Conway, *Medical and Legal Views of Death: Confrontation and Reconciliation,* 19 St. Louis U.L.J. 172 (1974). Arent, *The Criteria for Determining Death in Vital Organ Transplants – A Medical-Legal Dilemma,* 38 Mo. L. Rev. 220 (1973); Biorck, *When is Death?,* 1968 Wis. L. Rev. 484; Black, *Brain Death, Part I,* 299 N. Eng. J. Med. 393 (1978); Cantor, *Quinlan, Privacy, and the Handling of Incompetent Dying Patients* 30 Rutgers L. Rev. 243 (1977); Collestar, Jr., *Death, Dying and the Law: A Prosecutorial View of the Quinlan Case,* 30 Rutgers L. Rev. 304 (1977); Frederick II, *Medical Jurisprudence – Determining The Time of Death of the Heart Transplant Donor,* 51 N.C.L. Rev. 172 (1972); Friloux, Jr., *Death, When Does it Occur?,* 27 Baylor L. Rev. 10 (1975); Hirsh, *Brain Death,* 1975 Med. Trial Tech. Q. 377; Hoffman and Van Cura, *Death – The Five Brain Criteria,* 1978 Med. Trial Tech. Q. 377; Note, *The Tragic*

Choice; Termination of Care for Patients in a Permanent State, 51 N.Y.U.L. Rev. 285 (1976). Wasmuth, Jr., *The Concept of Death,* 30 Ohio St. L. Rev. 32 (1969). *Refinements in Criteria for the Determination of Death: An Appraisal,* 221 J.A.M.A. 48 (1972). *An Appraisal of the Criteria of Cerebral Death, A Summary Statement,* 237 J.A.M.A. 982 (1977). Capron and Kass, *A Statutory Definition of the Standards for Determining Human Death: An Appraisal and a Proposal,* 121 U. Penn L. Rev. 87 (1972). For an excellent review of this subject see: VanTill, A., *Diagnosis of Death in Comatose Patients under Resuscitation Treatment: A Critical Review of the Harvard Report,* 2 Am. Jour. Law and Med. 1-40 (1976). See also Veith, F. et al., *Brain Death,* 238 J.A.M.A. 1651-1655 (1977) and 238 J.A.M.A. 1744-1748 (1977); Byrne et al., *Brain Death – An Opposing Viewpoint,* 242 J.A.M.A. 1985-1990 (1979); *Editorial,* 242 J.A.M.A. 2001, 2002 (1979); Horan and Mall, *Death, Dying and Euthanasia,* University Publications of America, Inc., Washington, D.C., 1977.

4. Under the common law a person was considered dead when there was "total stoppage of the circulation of the blood, and a cessation of the animal and vital functions consequent thereon, such a respiration, pulsation, etc.," *Black's Law Dictionary* (4th ed. 1951), p. 488.

5. The common law can be interpreted broadly enough to include permanent cessation of brain functions as one of the definitions of death. One of the common law definitions of death was "cessation of life," *Bouvier's Law Dictionary* (Rawle's ed.), p. 775 (1914); *Cyclopedic Law Dictionary,* p. 285 (1922).

6. Olinger, S.D., *Medical Death,* 1 Baylor L. Rev. 22-26 (1975) (the entire issue of this law review is devoted to the issue of euthanasia).

7. See, e.g., Editorial of J.A.M.A., Nov. 2, 1979, Vol. 242, No. 18, pp. 2001, 2002 where Robert M. Veatch, Ph.D. says: "But the historical evolution has slowed. While approximately 20 states have adopted legal changes in the years after the Harvard report, the rate of change has recently decreased. Physicians are, or should be, bound by law. Where the definitions of death has not been changed, newer criteria for death pronouncement based on brain function should not be used."

8. See the discussion in: Ramsey, Paul, *The Patient as Person* (New Haven & London: Yale University Press, 1979).

9. Op. cit. ft. 1.

10. Capron & Kass, op. cit. ft. 3 at pp. 108-111.

11. Ramsey, op. cit. ft. 8 at p. 101.

12. Op. cit. ft. 2.

13. 366 N.E. 2d 744 (Sup. Ct. Mass, 1977).

14. 367 N.Y.S.2d 686 (1975).

15. *Lovato et al. v. District Court, et al.,* Supreme Court of Colorado, N. 79 SA 407 dec. 10-15-79. Slip Opinion.

16. Ibid. p. 20.

17. Uniform Brain Death Act drafted by the National Conference of Commissioners on Uniform State Laws, approved at its annual conference July 28 – August 4, 1978. The Commissioners appended two comments to the act, the second of which states: " 'Functioning' is a critical word in the Act. It expresses the idea of purposeful activity in all parts of the brain, as distinguished from random activity. In a dead brain, some meaningless cellular processes, detectable by sensitive monitoring equipment, could create legal confusion if the word 'activity' were substituted for functioning." The comment is unfortunate and detracts from the usefulness of the Act. It states that measurable activity of the brain which can be detected by sensitive monitoring equipment would not deter the diagnosis of brain death if the activity were meaningless cellular activity. The EEG detects only cortical activity. If this is the sensitive equipment referred to, then the Uniform Commissioners have unwittingly contradicted an almost universally accepted minimal sign of brain death: a flat EEG. This is probably not what was meant but no further explanation is offered by the Commissioners. The comment seems most inappropriate and confusing. States which adopted the Uniform Brain Death Act are urged *not* to adopt the Commissioners' comments and even requested in their legislative history to explicitly repudiate the comments. The important language of the UBDA ("sustained irreversible cessation of all functioning of the brain, including the brain stem, is dead") is adequate, stands on its own two feet and needs no gloss which seems to repudiate the meaning of the words used in the Act itself.

The UBDA states that the determination of death can be made according to "reasonable medical standards." This also is an unfortunate choice of words. Most brain death acts apply the correct phraseology of "customary medical standards," meaning that the medical profession itself sets the standard by determining what is customary in medical practice. This is the usual method of determining standards under Tort law. There are cases which adopt a reasonable rather than customary standard, *Helling v. Carey,* 83 Wash. 514 (1974). But such cases represent a decided deviation from the norm. Why the Commissioners should accept language setting a standard so at odds with what is legally acceptable under current standards is hard to understand.

18. Horan, D.J., *Euthanasia and Brain Death: Ethical and Legal Considerations,* 315 Annals of the New York Academy of Sciences 363-375 (1978).

19. That the diagnosis may be medically difficult to make is made clear by Volume 315 of the Annals of the New York Academy of Sciences, the entire volume of which is devoted to the subject of brain death on a medical, scientific, legal and moral basis.

20. *An Appraisal of the Criteria of Cerebral Death,* 237 J.A.M.A. 982-986 (1977).

21. Byrne et al., *Brain Death – An Opposing Viewpoint,* 242 J.A.M.A. 1985-1990 (1979).

22. See, Van Till, op. cit. ft. 3 at pp. 8-12. In his rebuttal editorial to the Byrne article Veatch praises the Byrne article as a challenge to be more precise in specifying what it is whose irreversible loss signals death of the person.

23. Horan, op. cit. ft. 18.

Theological and Pastoral Implications of Brain Death

Reverend Thomas J. O'Donnell, S.J.

Man's concept of death has a history as long and as varied as the history of mankind itself. Doubtless from the moment that Eve, the mother of all the living, held the dead body of Abel in her arms, men have always been baffled by the mystery of death. Frustrated by its inevitability and shocked into stark terror or dumb submission by the thought of no longer being alive, mortal man resorts to an almost universal experience. Thus do we pull a sheet over the face of a corpse so as not to look upon the face of death and blithely refer to our public records of death as "vital statistics."

James Gutmann of Columbia has observed that contemporary philosophical analysts are disposed to reject "unanswerable" questions as meaningless. Indeed, without the vision of faith and the guiding consolation of those words of the Lord: "I go to prepare a place for you" (John 14:3), many of today's philosophical attempts to define death beyond the most simple observations can quickly become esoteric exercises in futility. An example is Robert Morison's life-death-continuum concept.

An unprejudiced look at the biological facts suggests, indeed, that the life of a complex vertebrate like man is not a clearly defined entity with sharp discontinuities at both ends. On the contrary, the living human being starts inconspicuously, and at an unknown time, with the conjugation of two haploid cells.

And earlier in the same article he writes:

Death is no more a single, clearly delimited, momentary phenomenon than is infancy, adolescence, or middle age. The gradualness of the process of dying is even clearer than it was in Shakespeare's time, for we now know that various parts of the body can go on living for months after its central organization has disintegrated. Some cell lines, in fact, can be continued indefinitely.[1]

From there Morison moves to a "quality of life" criterion which equates might-as-well-be dead (in whose estimation is not clear) with being-dead. And he further complicates the problem by admitting that he cannot see the moral difference between what is today called negative and positive euthanasia, since the intention appears to be the same in the two cases. This, of course, is a common enough difficulty for those who recognize *finis operantis* (motive) as the total finality of any human action and reject the notion of *finis operis* (the nature of the act). But, as Leon Kass points out, the agent of death in negative euthanasia (not using extraordinary means to prolong life) is the patient's disease, whereas the agent of death in positive euthanasia is the patient's physician.[2]

As for Morison's continuum, Kass points out how obviously erroneously it is conceived. And, we might add, even if it had a foundation in theory, it would be solved, in fact *moriendo* (if not *ambulando*).

So much for the esoteric. Our concerns are much more incarnational – or, in the context of the Catholic faith and modern medicine, down-to-earth-doctrinal, or: "What are we to think of 'brain death' when the question does come up?"

Historical Review of Church Law Concerning Time of Death

While Catholic teaching on the theological significance of death has been long and consistent (explicitly from the Council of Carthage in 418 to Vatican II), there has been little taught on the recognition or determination of the moment of death.

The standard canonical and moral authors of the present century, in commenting on the sacrament of the anointing of the sick (especially in regard to CIC 941, which deals with conditional administration of the sacrament) have usually drawn a distinction between "real" death and "apparent" death in terms of speculation as to when the soul (*anima intellectiva, principium vitae humanae, forma hominis*) is no longer present after the individual has been declared clinically (medically) dead. The implication of this distinction was summarized in one well known commentary as follows:

> In cases of previous illness and gradual weakening of the vitality, it is generally believed that the space of time between apparent death and actual dissolution is very short. In cases of sudden collapse in accidents, strokes of apoplexy, and the like, some writers hold that even two hours after the last signs of life extreme unction may be given conditionally.[3]

Some authors, rather arbitrarily it would seem, established such time limits as up to one-half hour at the close of a lingering illness, and up to even three hours after sudden death.

When, subsequent to Vatican II, the Congregation for Divine Worship prepared a new "Rite of Anointing and Pastoral Care of the Sick" (which Pope Paul VI promulgated by his Apostolic Constitution, *Sacram Unctionem Infirmorum,* Nov. 30, 1972) there was a change, at least in the collocation of ideas. Whereas canon 941 had dealt with various circumstances or doubts for conditional anointing (attained use of reason, real danger of death, actual death), number 15 of the new rite deals only with the question of death, in the following words:

> 15. When a priest has been called to attend a person who is already dead, he should pray for the dead person, asking that God forgive his sins and graciously receive him into his kingdom. The priest is not to administer the sacrament of anointing. But if the priest is doubtful whether the sick person is dead, he may administer the sacrament conditionally.

There was no further comment which might be related to the moment of death, either in the apostolic constitution itself or in the press conference by Monsignor A. G. Martimort on the occasion of its publication (Jan. 18, 1973). And it is interesting to note that Nicholas Halligan, O.P., in commenting on the new rite, retains the same time span for conditional anointing after apparent (or clinical) death as did the older authors.[4]

On the other hand, what has been viewed as the somewhat more direct language and the different collocation of ideas in the new rite has given rise to the general and approved pastoral practice of not taking the vague question of when the soul actually leaves the body as a norm for when to administer the sacrament conditionally. Indeed in *Study Text II, Anointing and Pastoral Care of the Sick,* published by the Bishops' Committee on the Liturgy,[5] we find the following:

> What about this *misleading* practice of anointing the apparent dead? The ritual clearly states that priests summoned to attend a person already dead are not to anoint, but are to pray for the deceased. Only if unsure whether the sick person is actually dead is the priest to anoint conditionally. [Emphasis added.]

Thus the theological concept of "apparent" death, while retaining its speculative validity, seems to have very little recognized practical application to present pastoral practice with regard to the anointing of the sick, in what is at least a semi-official context. (The various committees of the United States Catholic Conference do not speak officially for the body of the bishops, but their publications are routinely referred to the Committee on Doctrine and at least implicitly accepted by the conference.) And aside from the time-span for conditional anointing, it is difficult to see any practical application of the concept of "apparent" death. The theological concept of "apparent death" is equivalent to the medical-legal concept of definitive "clinical death," and it seems evident from a moral viewpoint that one would not need to delay such procedures as autopsy or the removal of organs for transplant just because, although the patient has been declared dead, the soul might not yet have left the body. It would be difficult to imagine how such procedures could be viewed either as hastening that exitus, or be in any way inappropriate or disrespectful.

With all this in mind, it is important to note five points made by Pope Pius XII in the most significant papal teaching that we have on the subject of the moment of death.[6] The Pope pointed out, among other things, that:

1. In doubt about the fact of death having occurred "it will be necessary to presume that life remains because there is involved here a fundamental right received from the Creator, and it is necessary to prove with certainty that it has been lost";

2. There is a difference between "human life" and "the simple life of organs";

3. There is a validity to the notion of "complete and final separation of the soul from the body, but in practice one must take into account the lack of precision of the terms 'body' and 'separation'";

4. General observation suggests that human life continues as long as the vital processes (distinguished from the simple life of organs) manifest themselves spontaneously "or even with the help of artificial processes." (In view of what follows it is important to note that Pius XII made this statement a decade before the concept and criteria of brain death began to be as carefully examined as in, and subsequent to, the Harvard criteria.)

5. Finally, in answer to the question of the moment of death (on or off the respirator) the Pope responded: "It remains for the doctor, and especially the anesthesiologist, to give a clear and precise definition of 'death' and the 'moment of death' of a patient who passes away in a state of unconsciousness." When asked, under the same circumstances of artificial resuscitation, "at what time does the Catholic Church consider the patient 'dead' or when must he be declared dead according to natural law?" the Pope responded: "Where the verification of the fact in particular cases is concerned, the answer cannot be deduced from any religious or moral principle and, under this aspect, does not fall within the competence of the Church. Until an answer can be given, the question must remain open."

These points have been selected from the allocution because, although not occurring in the same order as we have listed them here, they do, in this order, give us a summary of Catholic teaching on the moment of death.

The Roman Pontiff left the matter primarily to the judgment of the physicians. Thus likewise, in *The Ethical and Religious Directives for Catholic Health Facilities*[7] the same teaching is stated in directive 31: "Post-mortem examinations must not be begun until death is morally certain. Vital organs, that is, organs necessary to sustain life, may not be removed until death has taken place. The determination of the time of death must be made in accordance with responsible and commonly accepted scientific criteria. . . ."

What remains to be done in this study is to align the current scientific and medical criteria for judging the moment of death with these concepts drawn from Catholic teaching, and to make some comments where indicated.

Other Definitions of Death

What "death" means in the common estimate of men is adequately reflected, in simple terms, in the *Webster New Collegiate Dictionary* (1977): "the permanent cessation of all vital functions: the end of life." *Dorland's Medical Dictionary* (25th– and currently latest– edition, 1965) similarly defines death as: "the cessation of life; permanent cessation of all vital bodily functions." This is an obvious reference to those signs which have always been easily identifiable (the permanent cessation of respiration, heart beat and circulation) until the advent of mechanical resuscitators began to mask the usual symptoms of death in some cases. Thus the dictionary significantly adds:

> For legal and medical purposes, the following definition of death has been proposed – the irreversible cessation of all of the following (1) total cerebral function, (2) spontaneous function of the respiratory system, and (3) spontaneous function of the circulatory system.

This proposal is essentially an early summary of the criteria for total brain death, without the mention of the confirmatory evidence of the flat encephalogram under certain specified conditions (such as the ruling out of deep hypothermia or deep barbiturate poisoning, which may produce a temporary flat encephalogram).

It might also be noted, in passing, that *Dorland's Medical Dictionary,* among the other subdivisions of the word "death," defines "apparent death" in the obvious sense of apparent *only* (and not in the theological sense of the term as we have seen it) as: "a state of complete interruption of bodily processes from which the patient can be resuscitated." There is also the contrasting of "somatic death" as the "cessation of all vital cellular activity" with "local death" as "death of a part of the body," or what we would rather call "necrosis" of specified tissue or groups of cells.

For our purposes it is most important to note that, among *Dorland's* subdivisions of the word "death," we find "brain death" referred to as "irreversible coma." It is most important to note and comment on this because here we have an unusual and misleading use of the word "coma." To most people, coma means a state of unconsciousness from which the (living) patient cannot be aroused.

And this is likewise the medically accepted meaning of "coma" and indeed is the definition of "coma" (under its own listing) in the dictionary itself. But any concept of brain death as merely irreversible coma inevitably leads to confusion. As Dr. William Sweet has pointed out recently in a distinguished medical journal:

> . . . it is essential that a clear distinction be made between death of the brain and a prolonged or irreversible state of coma but with some evidence of brain-related bodily function. Not only are the two terms not synonymous, but they describe two different states that do not overlap. Once a person is dead, he is no longer in coma . . . Indeed, it is clear that the brain does not die all at once, and the "coma" sense of "brain death" could mean rather only the necrosis of some parts of the brain (such as the cortex). By "brain death" in the sense of "real death" we mean "total brain death," or the death of the entire brain and central nervous system.[8]

Later in his editorial, Dr. Sweet makes the following astute observation:

> . . . it is clear that a person is not dead *unless* his brain is dead. The time-honored criteria of stoppage of the heartbeat and circulation are indicative of death only when they persist long enough for the brain to die.

In addition to the confirmatory evidence of the flat electroencephalogram (under the conditions mentioned above), the absence of cerebral circulation as demonstrated by isotope angiography has been viewed as confirmatory of brain death. This results in "a characteristic softened and liquified appearance at autopsy" that occurs "when cerebral circulatory arrest results from increased cranial pressure and changes in the brain microvascular circulation while body temperature and other functions are preserved."[9]

These medical observations are repeated here for information, and not for scientific evaluation. The latter remains within the competence of the medical and scientific communities. The theological conclusion that seems to be warranted is that if and when (if not already) the competent and responsible sectors of the medical and scientific communities agree upon and accept neurological criteria for definitive clinical death, the theological community may accept these criteria as valid and operative in determining that death has occurred. Then we could conclude that the one-time patient on the respirator becomes, at that point, a mechanically perfused cadaver.

Notes

1. R. S. Morison, "Death: Process or Event?" *Science,* August 1971, pp. 694-698.

2. Leon R. Kass, "Death As an Event: A Comment on Robert Morison," *Science,* August 1971, pp. 698-702.

3. Stanislaus Woywood, O.F.M., *A Practical Commentary on the Code of Canon Law,* revised by Callistus Smith, O.F.M. (New York: Herder, 1957), p. 549.

4. N. Halligan, O.P., *The Ministry of the Concelebration of the Sacraments* (Staten Island: Alba House, 1973), II:205.

5. Washington, D.C.: U.S. Catholic Conference, 1973, p. 10.

6. Allocution to an International Congress of Anesthesiologists, November 24, 1957.

7. Approved by the United States National Conference of Catholic Bishops, November 1971.

8. William H. Sweet, M.D., "Brain Death" (editorial), *The New England Journal of Medicine,* August 24, 1978.

9. J. M. Goodman, M.D., and L. L. Heck, M.D., *Journal of the American Medical Association,* August 29, 1977, pp. 966-68.

Introduction to Prolonging Life Issues

Reverend Donald G. McCarthy, Ph.D.

In our society we have a consensus, both religious and secular, that human life has an inherent, existential value, and that this value precedes the functional value individuals achieve in their human activity. Of course, we do not exist or develop alone but in society. The community of our human relationships offers each of us the setting in which our physical experience becomes humanized and our temporal experience opens out to the transcendent.

Secular language about human life does not use the word "sanctity" but "dignity." We recognize universal human dignity in documents like the United Nations' Universal Declaration of Human Rights. The term "inherent dignity" is a beautiful term because it means our dignity inheres within us, it sticks to our bones. There is a real question whether the secular term "dignity of human life" adequately supports "morally equal" human dignity in a totally horizontal perspective without transcendence. When we look to establish that morally equal dignity we look to the meaning of human life which transcends the material or physical meaning.

The religious language of "sanctity of human life" relates to theological concepts like the Fatherhood of God, and, in Christian belief, the redemption of all people by Jesus Christ. There is no questioning here of the morally equal dignity of all human persons which is strongly supported by the religious perspective of equality under God.

We can summarize the community values that we observe with regard to the dignity and sanctity of human life. The first principle which has been honored by civilized nations is that one must not destroy innocent human life. The human equality principle is the secular principle supporting this even though it may not have an incontestable base in a philosophy which excludes transcendence. The sanctity of life principle supports this as a religious or theistic principle.

The prolonging life issues which face society today are often summarized by suggesting that prolonging life must be distinguished from prolonging death. Before such issues can be faced, however, the use of the term "passive euthanasia" must be reviewed.

The Terminology of Passive Euthanasia

The Webster 1977 dictionary definition of euthanasia describes it as an act or practice of killing individuals. This has often been described as voluntary or involuntary depending on whether the individual wishes to be killed.

"Passive euthanasia" is the term which is creating confusion. It has been used by the organization now called Concern for Dying (formerly the Euthanasia Educational Council) which has been associated with the Society for the Right to Die (formerly the Euthanasia Society of America). This term's definition simply speaks of "an act or omission requested by the patient" with no distinction of what is being omitted. It could be the omission of food, of a respirator, or of anything. Death occurs after this omission and, since there is no act of killing, the term "passive euthanasia" is being used.

An older description of passive euthanasia speaks of it as "inducing a peaceful death by omission of life-prolonging efforts." Here there is an implication of "death control" and, again, there is no distinction of what kind of omission may precede the death.

Hence this terminology suggests that active euthanasia describes acts of killing and passive euthanasia describes all cases of allowing to die. This, of course, raises the question of, when is it morally acceptable to allow someone to die? If we omit ordinary efforts to prolong life, in the Catholic tradition at least, that is homicide by omission or criminal negligence. The omission of extraordinary efforts, however, may be justifiable. I have coined a phrase to indicate this possibility: "Justifiable Use of Conservative Therapy Only" (JUCTO). This describes the case of what the Catholic tradition would call the omitting of ethically extraordinary means of prolonging life. We have said in this tradition that something is *ethically* extraordinary if it does not offer reasonable hope of benefit or involves excess pain, expense, or other hardship. Medicine may use these terms in a different sense so that a procedure may be "medically ordinary" but "ethically extraordinary."

The "reasonable hope of benefit" which makes a procedure "ethically" ordinary is a very difficult question. We can agree that a reasonable hope of benefit does not exist when death is imminent or when we have a medically certain irreversible coma as in the case of Karen Quinlan. She was removed from the respirator because it was considered "ethically extraordinary."

Within the Catholic tradition the omission of an "ethically" extraordinary means of prolonging life has not been considered morally objectionable. But the omission of an "ethically" ordinary means is considered morally objectionable and equivalent to the act of killing.

The problem with the term "passive euthanasia," then, is that it covers any and all forms of omission and admits of the active intention to induce death. If we used circles to represent the extent of application of terms, "passive euthanasia" would be represented by a large circle (indicating all the possible omissions) and "JUCTO" would be a small circle within the larger one. Hence we can give examples of forms of passive euthanasia which would be immoral in the Catholic tradition of respect for life, falling outside the small circle but within the larger one.

Hence, I present a slogan, "loose terms lose values." The use of the loose term "passive euthanasia" can gloss over the very different ethical status of omissions which may precede death. One could summarize the objections to this euthanasia terminology by saying that active euthanasia is a redundant term because the simple word "euthanasia" already means active killing. On the other hand, the term passive euthanasia, because it covers all forms of omissions, is an incoherent term and it loses our respect for the necessary care that we are obliged to provide others by love of neighbor and the Gospel.

Managing Pain and Prolonging Life

Vincent J. Collins, M.D.

Analysis of Pain and Suffering

Pain and suffering are experienced by everyone, and each has had a good share by the time we reach fifty years of age if not long before. I think that a pain-free society is a fantasy. However, I would like to analyze pain and suffering and its relief from the perspective of a physician who deals with a great deal of pain in the clinic setting.

First, let us define pain. Our working definition of pain is that it is an experience. When we analyze this experience, it is found to have two components. We recognize a physiological component which provides the means by which sensation reaches the brain and is perceived. The sequence is somewhat as follows. Stimuli are applied to various parts of the body; specifically, when we touch something extremely hot, we respond very appropriately. The hot stimulus is carried as an impulse by specific nerves over a set of pathways to a specific area of the lower part of the brain or the subcortex of the brain, called the thalamus. There are also pathways to carry pain from viscera. Thus, there are two separate pathways, one to carry cutaneous and special senses and the other to carry deeper or organ sensations. The physiological component is the perception element.

The second component is the psychological one. This is the analysis system for the processing of sensory information at higher brain centers. With regard to the psychological component, it is the appreciative element; it analyzes and quantitates each sensation, it integrates such things as our memory, past experiences, our mood effect, the kinds of emotional overlays that might exist, problems that have faced society in trying to alleviate pain.

Definition of Euthanasia

Now with that I would like to then proceed to a subject that is so important that you and we, all together, must fight against its application. The subject is euthanasia. Euthanasia has been put forth as a means for our society to relieve suffering. It is, of course, in its ultimate value, a destruction of life. We destroy the sufferer in order to relieve the suffering. That, of course, is anathema to a good physician. I then ask the question – why euthanasia? What is the need? We have intimated that the answer proposed is to relieve suffering; and that is indeed the argument employed by those who are pro-euthanasia. It is a good cause, indeed, to relieve suffering, but the means is, of course, totally inimical to the profession of medicine (and to society), which is to save life, not to do any harm. *Primum non nocere* is still a guideline for our practice.

Father Donald McCarthy pointed out (see pp. 141-143) that "active" euthanasia is a redundant term. Euthanasia stands by itself – it needs no qualification. The definition is clear, not only in modern dictionaries, but traditionally and historically from the Greeks on down. It has been understood to be an act: a positive act of commission. Furthermore, we must disabuse society of the use of the adjective "passive" applied to euthanasia. There is no such thing; it is a total contradiction in terms. Euthanasia by definition is an action.

Conditions Advocated by Euthanasia Proponents

But, there are certain conditions, of course, that euthanasia proponents lay down before one decides to end a life, to kill a suffering person. What are these conditions that are laid down? The first is: an incurable illness. We will accept that there are disease states

145

for which we do not have a cure. But, if we say that there is no help for the sufferer and no prospect of aid, this I will deny and most physicians will deny it. There are help and strategies for relieving pain.

Secondly, we do recognize that there is intolerable pain, but we also will say that there is no such thing as intractable pain. I deny that there is any kind of a pain situation which we cannot in some way or another relieve. And I would point out that at the present time throughout at least this country and in England and a few other Western countries and even in Russia, physicians and others are developing what are called Pain Control Centers. Such clinics were conceived by Dr. Rovenstien at Bellevue Hospital. And, indeed, in New York, we established a nerve block clinic at St. Vincent's Hospital. It flourished and I believe that it is still active.

A third condition proposed for euthanasia is that there is an expressed rational desire to die. I do not believe that anyone who is suffering intensely, has an intense physical or mental pain, can make a rational decision and deliberately ask to be killed. A person may say, "I wish I were dead," but the wishing and the actual asking that someone, much less a physician, go ahead and kill him is unlikely and I have really not encountered such patients.

Character of Euthanasia

But, what is the character of euthanasia? Here are some of its features. It is absolutely not therapeutic. It doesn't improve the patient's life or benefit the patient in any way. It is an action by another person that causes death. It is misguided mercy at best. It does involve a harm. Whatever method used would result in total disfunction. It also would be destructive to all organs of the body. If a lethal dose of a depressant drug or an anesthetic agent, and/or a paralytic agent were administered to a patient, it would certainly not be beneficial or therapeutic. What then does euthanasia amount to? It amounts to the abandonment of the patient, and that is the sum and substance. It is a form of exterminative medicine.

We have said that mercy killing is anathema and undesirable in our society because it opens up a Pandora's box of what we can possibly do to control the various ills that afflict our society and to determine the fate of those who may not have value, at least in the eyes of some. We have an alternative which is really a restatement of the traditional ethical practice of medicine. It is termed "therapeutic

146

rationalism."

Let's examine the basis upon which medicine and surgical treatment rests. There are indications and there are contra-indications to all forms of therapy – drug or procedure. The indications are that we use appropriate treatment. For example, we do not use digitalis to treat diabetes. We do not use insulin to treat heart failure. These are inappropriate drugs for those conditions. Their use here is irrational and non-therapeutic. That, of course, mechanically speaking, is a ridiculous situation, a point, but it emphasizes what we are speaking about. If any measure is inappropriate, or if indeed we have used an appropriate measure, but it is not effective, it is not bringing a person back either to an acceptable level of function or improving the individual, then we have a right to choose some other type of therapeutic measure and discontinue using the one at hand. This discontinuing of ineffective therapy – a drug or a procedure such as surgery or a life support in irreversible coma or brain death – whether rational therapeutics or therapeutic rationalism, is appropriate treatment.

Strategies to Relieve Pain

Let us examine again the problem of intolerable pain and intolerable suffering. Yes, it exists, but I again emphasize that today we have many strategies that enable us to make it tractable – we can indeed relieve pain and suffering. What are these strategies? There are several principal categories. We can remove the stimulus; you will do it automatically when you hit the hot stove – you immediately remove your finger from the hot stove; it is withdrawal of the painful stimulus. We can remove various kinds of stimuli, for example, in a patient with a growing tumor that is pressing against a nerve and causing pain. We can reduce the size of the tumor by radiation or reduce the size by means of chemotherapeutic agents or remove the tumor by surgery. When the compression of the nerve is eliminated, that pain ceases.

Secondly, if the previous procedures are impractical, we can block the sensory nerves. Every sensory nerve passes from the periphery of the body to the brain up through the spinal cord, through the thalamic area to the cortex. At various steps along the way, the nerve can either be blocked by an anesthetic or chemically destroyed. Pain fibers can be selectively destroyed without paralyzing a patient. We can do that today. We have over 300 patients who have had cancer of the cervix and who have had a spread of the cancer to the pelvic organs and to the hips. In most instances, these patients have been on high doses of morphine and other narcotic drugs. We have identified the nerves by doing differential anesthesia. Having identified the nerves with an ordinary local anesthetic, novocain type, we have then proceeded to administer small amounts of absolute alcohol, small volumes, and destroyed those pain nerves specifically. These patients have gone home and died at home, pain free, in the bosom of their families. This can be done.

There are many other strategies, such as raising the pain threshold by use of analgesic drugs. This is the category in which most of our drugs fall: morphine, methadone and demerol; they fall into the category of raising the pain threshold at the thalamic level as well as inhibiting the experience of pain at certain cortical levels where the projection of the sense input from the thalamus goes before it is appreciated.

Neuro-psychological techniques are available to relieve pain. Psychologically, we can provide sympathy, care and compassion, we can suffer with the patient. After all, that's what compassion really is — sharing ourselves with the sufferer.

Pharmacologically, we have sedatives, we even have used LSD with good purpose in small doses. Hallucinogens flood the individual with all kinds of good sensations in a set environment so that the pain is blotted out.

Medically, we have the chemotherapeutic means; we can provide a regimen of general conditioning of the body so that the person is able to cope with pain more effectively. Another strategy is acupuncture. In selected cases, we have a few patients in whom the neurophysiologic and psychologic effects of acupuncture provide relief.

There are other techniques. We have biofeedback. We determine the pattern of brain waves when pain is under control and the circumstances that have produced this pattern. We try to have the patient reproduce those kinds of brain waves and condition himself to stop pain. We have hypnotherapy and music and hypnosis and general comfort; these are all neuro-psychological techniques. We use anti-depressant drugs. It is usual that a patient who has chronic pain feels depressed. If we elevate his mood he tolerates the pain much better. We also have the strategy of sending a patient home with a flask of an analgesic usually containing morphine. It is called the Brompton's Hospital mixture, since the original pharmaceutical preparation was made in London in Brompton Hospital. We have Slesinger's mixture in this country. Patients go home and can take their medication ad lib. We don't tell them every 2, 4, 8 hours. They take it whenever they want it. And the security of knowing that they have something available next to their bedside has an amazing beneficial effect. Patients are comforted by the presence of the available pain reliever and they cut down their dosage from what they have been taking to prove that particular point. Addiction is not a concern; indeed, it is not seen in the abuse sense and would be a small price to pay in terminal illness in order to relieve suffering.

There is one other problem that follows the matter of suffering. When a patient is in a terminal state, what do we do when a cardiac arrest occurs? There are several considerations if the cardiac arrest is related to an acute condition (drug, heart attack, hemorrhage) and CPR is instituted (resuscitation measures). Total care should be pursued. But, there are situations when it is obvious from the causative factors that one doesn't institute CPR when the heart stops. There are situations when no intensive care should be instituted at all: massive stroke, physiologic deterioration from advancing cancer, irreversible coma, massive coronary attack. Resuscitation should be determined by the expected outcome. This is rational therapeutics and ethically proper. To use extraordinary measures otherwise is bad medical practice and, indeed, immoral.

"Right to Die" Legislation: Current Legal Status

Dennis J. Horan, J.D.

In 1976 California became the first state to pass legislation dealing with the so-called Right to Die.[1] Such legislation is also referred to as living will legislation or natural death legislation. By 1977, seven other states had passed similar legislation.[2] Since then only two other states have done so, Kansas and Washington.[3] Texas and North Carolina have recently amended their statutes.[4] Generally speaking, such legislation allows a person to execute a directive to his physician for the purpose of withholding medical treatment at some later date, usually when the patient has reached a terminal state.

"Right to Die" Organizations

Because of the lobbying activities of such groups as the Society for the Right to Die similar legislation has been introduced and is pending in almost every state in the union.[5] The Society for the Right to Die is located at 250 West 57th Street in New York City, which is the same address as the organization now called Concern for the Dying which was formerly the Euthanasia Educational Council.

In 1938, the Euthanasia Society of America, predecessor of the Society for the Right to Die, was founded to legalize the right of incurable sufferers to a "good death."

In 1967, the "Living Will" was proposed at a meeting of the Euthanasia Society by Luis Kutner, a Chicago attorney and president of World Habeas Corpus.

In the same year, the Euthanasia Educational Fund (later the Euthanasia Educational Council and then Concern for Dying) was established by the Society's Board of Directors as a tax-deductible organization to undertake a program of public and professional education to further the goals of the Euthanasia Society.

In 1975, the Euthanasia Society of America became the Society for the Right to Die, assuming a leadership role as the only organization in the United States with a program dedicated to active support of "death with dignity" legislation.[6]

Although these organizations share many of the same board members, Concern for the Dying no longer funds the Society for the Right to Die. In recent correspondence to the Society, Concern for the Dying expressed its reasoning as follows:

> . . . there are markedly disparate outlooks and modes of operations on the part of the two Boards. *The Society's is an activist program crusading for a cause.* The Concern's is one of philosophic exploration of issues and their ramifications, based on the belief that the best form of teaching is to present all sides of a problem. . . . The Council Board has therefore come to the conclusion that it should hereby relinquish its responsibility for raising funds to support the Society and should release the Society from its agreement not to raise funds on its own behalf.[7]

In urging its members to continue to support its activist program, the Society indicates that in the 1980's it will press ahead with its legislative, judicial and educational programs. These programs are instructive and constitute the entire array of mechanisms for activist public policy impact and change. At the present time they are especially interested in achieving their aids through litigation as well as legislation and education.[8]

Both organizations applaud passage of the legislation we are considering here. Their ultimate goals probably include the legalization of assisted suicide, the creation of suicide centers and the full legalization of voluntary euthanasia both assisted and unassisted.

In some instances they would probably support the legalization of involuntary euthanasia with proper legal safeguards. They realize, however, that they cannot foist their ideas too strongly and too soon on a society not yet ready to consider them since they will thus damage if not destroy their effectiveness. By moving cautiously and without stridency they hope to gain a larger audience for their views.

The Executive Director of the Concern for the Dying organization has stated:

> On the subject of crisis centers for potential suicides, or the granting of access to lethal substances, we feel that the time is not yet right to take a public position. In fact, even within our own board of directors there is concern that potential abuses of changes in law in these areas must be further examined and avoidance mechanisms developed before we could actively support and encourage such changes.[9]

Concern for the Dying is also very active in support of the Hospice Movement.[10] Richard Lammerton has expressed his concern about the growing influence in America of Concern for the Dying in the Hospice Movement.[11] One can only wonder at the ultimate aim of these organizations in terms of their influence on Hospice. The interest of active supporters of euthanasia and suicide in Hospice makes one wonder what that interest is all about.

Some Aspects of Right to Die Legislation

In any event, these organizations have successfully created public policy changes in the wake of the *Quinlan* case by the passage of the ten right to die bills under consideration here. I have analyzed these bills elsewhere as to many of their deficiencies.[12] The primary deficiency I described as:

> Such legislation is likely to inhibit the physician's effort to treat the dying patient with dignity, grace and a measure of humanity in yet another way. Whenever a statute is enacted regulating conduct, especially where punitive sanctions are available for non-compliance, the effect is to chill and inhibit similar conduct otherwise legal but not now in conformity with the requirements of the act. Thus, physicians may be reluctant to withdraw or withhold life-sustaining treatment unless a directive has been executed by the patient, even though there is no legal obligation to extend heroic or useless care. If even twenty percent of the

population executed a living will within the requirements of the given statute – an optimistic figure in view of the small percentage who execute treatments for disposition of property – the remaining eighty percent must suffer the consequences. California attempted to mitigate this problem through Section 7193, which indicates that its "Natural Death Act" does not impair or supersede any prior right or responsibility the person possesses to effect the lawful withdrawal of life-sustaining procedures.[13]

Another aspect of concern, however, is whether this legislation promotes mercy killing or will lead to mercy killing. Yale Kamisar, Professor of Criminal Law at the University of Michigan Law School, in his famous article on mercy killing, writes about the history of the English Euthanasia Society and the American forerunners of the currently existing organizations. He outlines their ultimate aims and warns later in the article about the dangers of embarking on the slippery slope. One step onto that slope will lead to an uncontrollable slide into things we never thought could happen in our society.[14] One is tempted to say, just as we never thought abortion could ever be legal in our society.

Do these ten bills promote or will they help promote euthanasia or mercy killing? First of all, I should point out that these statutes are unnecessary, create more legal problems than they solve, do not aid the family or physician in solving the dying with dignity problem, are sometimes sloppily drafted, do not show an understanding of the nature of the problem – in short are legal abominations.[15] Some statutes, such as that of California, contain explicit language, even though unnecessary since euthanasia is a homicide under our law, that they are not legalizing mercy killing. This is good. In addition, the well-drafted statutes are limited to adults and are effective only in a truly terminal situation.

Examples of Legislation

For example, the California Act requires that the adult must be in a terminal condition before the directive to the physician is effective. Terminal condition is defined as an incurable condition caused by injury, disease or illness which, regardless of the application of life-sustaining procedures, would, within reasonable medical judgment, produce death, and where the application of life-sustaining procedures serves only to postpone the moment of death of the

153

patient. A life-sustaining procedure is defined to mean a procedure or intervention which utilizes mechanical or other artificial means to sustain, restore, or supplant a vital function, which, when applied to a qualified patient, would serve only to artificially prolong the moment of death and where, in the judgment of the attending physician, death is imminent whether or not such procedures are utilized. If such legislation is to be passed at all, these safeguards are essential since they keep the act within the proper standards of medical care and treatment in our society and are consistent with the values we seek to preserve. When truly limited to a terminal condition under the standards stated in the California Act such legislation, although unnecessary, does not violate any of the values we seek to preserve. Under these circumstances our concern must be to see that these safeguards are not changed by amendment.[16] However, other acts which have not been so carefully drafted do not contain these safeguards.

A classic example in this area of legislation gone berserk is the Arkansas Act.[17] Section one of the Act creates a right to die with dignity and to refuse medical treatment. The common law already gives the right to refuse medical treatment which is probably not as absolute as is usually thought but the exception need not deter us here.[18] The decision to reject medical treatment even in terminal cases when done by a competent adult cannot properly be construed as suicide or euthanasia,[19] and it is not a right that needs statutory authority.

Section two allows the creation of a directive to reject any "artificial, extraordinary, extreme or radical medical or surgical means or procedures calculated to prolong his life." Any hospital or physician who acts on the directive is immune from liability. The act does not state that the illness must be terminal, and does not define the words used: "artificial," "extraordinary," "extreme" or "radical."

Presumably since it is not limited, the act applies at any time and under any circumstances. It is so unlimited that one wonders what was in the mind of its sponsors. We do know that, of all ten such statutes, the Arkansas statute is the one most highly praised by the Society for the Right to Die. As a matter of fact, the Arkansas statute goes much further than the model bill of the Society for the Right to Die published in their 1976 legislative manual. Even that model bill is limited to adults and applies only to terminal illnesses.[20]

154

Section three of the Arkansas statute is an unbelievable approach to these problems. This section allows a parent or guardian to execute a directive for anyone, even a minor, who is mentally unable to execute one "or who is *otherwise* incapacitated." Needless to say, "otherwise incapacitated" is undefined in the act. The abuses capable under this act are beyond imagination. In addition, the act gives preferences as to who may execute the directive on behalf of another to the extent of allowing a majority of the children to do so if a spouse is unwilling or unable to act. Imagine the children taking a vote to determine whether medical means to prolong a parent's life should be used! Imagine a majority of the children voting to overrule a parent who is unwilling to execute the directive!

The Arkansas statute is an ill-conceived, ill-defined and sloppily drafted statute. It should be repealed. It is an unconstitutional withdrawal of the protection of life without due process or equal protection. It is tantamount to the legalization of euthanasia. It is this type of statute that illustrates the dangers in death legislation, which must be carefully monitored at every legislative level. If there must be such legislation, then effort must be made to ensure the necessary safeguards. Such legislation must be effective only in truly terminal cases; it must not allow withdrawal of sustenance or ordinary medical means; it must apply only to adults; it must not seek mandatory control over the physician's judgment; it must not require complex procedures, as are usually found in the probate court; it must ensure that consent was given voluntarily; it must prohibit euthanasia or mercy killing.

Withdrawal of treatment for the terminally ill does not need legislative support. Indeed, several of the acts under consideration here contain specific sections indicating that the execution or non-execution of a directive does not supersede any existing legal right or legal responsibility which any person may have to effect the withholding or nonuse of any medical treatment in any lawful manner.[21] Several recent cases have dealt with the withholding or withdrawal of medical treatment and have enunciated the applicable legal standards.

Some Recent Cases

The leading case, of course, is the much celebrated *Quinlan* case.[11] Karen Ann Quinlan was a 22-year-old woman who was brought, unconscious, to the hospital. She was placed on a respirator but remained in a comatose condition. Ultimately her father sought court approval of the withdrawal of Karen from the respirator over the objections of the attending physician and hospital. The Supreme Court of New Jersey held that the father was a proper guardian and that he was authorized to terminate the respirator treatment if he obtained the concurrence of the responsible attending physicians, who must conclude that there is no reasonable possibility of Karen's ever emerging from her present comatose condition to a cognitive, sapient state and if he obtained also the same type of agreement from a hospital ethics committee.

It should be remembered that the *Quinlan* case was litigated on the almost unsaid basis[23] that Karen was in a terminal state. That this proved to be a factual error is significant only to show how mortal judges and litigants are. For our considerations, however, the application of the principles involved usually requires that the patient under consideration be deemed to have reached the terminal state.

The *Quinlan* court based its decision on the right to refuse medical treatment which it found in the constitutional right of privacy under both the federal and New Jersey constitutions. The court held that Karen's right of privacy – her right to refuse medical treatment – could be asserted by her guardian and family on her behalf under the particular circumstances of this case.[24] The court also concluded that these matters in the future could be handled by the family, the physician and the hospital ethics committee without application to a court.

The second most important case in this area of the law, while agreeing to most of what the *Quinlan* court said, severely criticized it for not requiring that all such decisions to withhold or withdraw treatment be made by a court of competent jurisdiction.

The *Saikewicz*[25] case involved a 67-year-old man with an I.Q. of 10 who had been institutionalized all his life and who had contracted acute myeloblastic monocytic leukemia for which the usual treatment is chemotherapy. The institution petitioned the court for a guardian to make the necessary decision. The guardian and the attending physicians recommended against the chemotherapy and the Supreme Court of Massachusetts ultimately affirmed this decision.

Once again, the *Saikewicz* court treated this as a case involving a terminal patient. Indeed, between the entry of its first order of

156

affirmance and the publication of its opinion 18 months passed, during which time Mr. Saikewicz "died without pain or discomfort."[26]

The *Saikewicz* court agreed with the New Jersey Supreme Court that Mr. Saikewicz's constitutional right of privacy was applicable. In addition, it felt that the best interests of the incompetent were to be considered and that this proved substituted judgment could be applied to the facts of the case. In affirming the guardian's decision not to treat, the court seemed to lean heavily on the inability of anyone with an I.Q. of 10 to comprehend and cooperate with the onerous and difficult treatment of chemotherapy. The court did criticize the *Quinlan* court for allowing family and physicians to make such decisions and did explicitly state that court approval of such decisions must be sought. This aspect of the decision has been severely criticized[27] and its importance minimized by the *Dinnerstein* decision.[28]

In *Saikewicz* the trial judge had agreed with the guardian's decision not to treat on the basis of the patient's (1) age, (2) inability to cooperate, (3) adverse side effects, (4) low chance of remissions, (5) suffering caused by chemotherapy, and (6) his quality of life remaining. The Supreme Court of Massachusetts agreed with the first five reasons but rejected any quality-of-life consideration in these cases. The court did give legal recognition to the distribution between ordinary and extra-ordinary treatment.

The *Saikewicz* court stated that the state's interest in such a patient is limited to (1) the preservation of life, (2) protecting the interests of innocent third parties, (3) the prevention of suicide and (4) the maintenance of ethical integrity of the medical profession. It found none of these conditions existing in this case and therefore ruled that the state had no intervening interest here.

The court limited the application of the *Saikewicz* rule, namely, that treatment may be withheld, to those cases where the patient has (1) an incurable and terminal illness, (2) where there exists no life saving or life-prolonging treatment, or (3) where the treatment would only effect a brief and uncertain delay in the natural death process.

It posits these as the applicable legal standards: (1) There exists in all persons a right to reject medical treatment under appropriate circumstances, (2) this right extends to an incompetent, (3) and may be exercised on his behalf when it is in his best interests, (4) but those best interests may not include quality-of-life consideration.

157

The court was quick to reject quality-of-life considerations stating that:

> ... the chance of a longer life carries the same weight for Saikewicz as for any other person, the value of life under law having no relation to intelligence or social positions.[29]

The uproar created by the requirement in *Saikewicz* that court approval be sought for any decision to withhold treatment quickly caused a Massachusetts appellate court to temper such a harsh rule by the application of common sense. In *Dinnerstein,*[30] it was held that court approval need not be sought unless life-saving or life-prolonging treatment alternatives are available and the decision was against use of those treatments. Where the case presents a question within the competence of the medical profession as to what measures are appropriate to ease the imminent passing of an irreversibly, terminally ill patient in light of her history and family wishes, that question is one not for judical decision but one for the attending physician. The court should only become involved if there is a contention that the physician failed to exercise the necessary degree of skill and competence.[31]

These decisions should be contrasted with the decision of the Supreme Court of Massachusetts in the famous *Chad Green* case.[32] Chad, at age 20 months, contracted leukemia. His parents refused to give him the appropriate treatment which was chemotherapy. The Supreme Court of Massachusetts affirmed a lower court decision taking custody from Chad's parents for the purpose of giving him chemotherapy. The court distinguished *Saikewicz* because here the treatment being withheld was both life-prolonging and life-saving. Under these circumstances the state's interest in protecting life overrides the parents' rights to direct the medical treatment of their child. The child's best interests also militate against non-treatment. For these reasons the court took custody from the parents for the purpose of requiring treatment.

So too, in the baby *Houle*[33] case the court appointed a guardian to give consent for surgical correction of a tracheal esophageal fistula of a five-day-old infant whose parents refused consent.

A review of these and other similar decisions teaches that medical treatment may be withdrawn by a physician when in his medical judgment it is useless. He is not mandated by the law to render useless treatment, nor does the standard of medical care require useless treatment.

By "useless" is meant that the continued use of the therapy cannot and does not improve the prognosis for recovery. Even if the therapy is necessary to maintain stability, such therapy should not be mandatory where the ultimate prognosis is hopeless. This does not mean that ordinary means of life supports, such as food and drink, can be discontinued merely because the ultimate prognosis is hopeless. It does mean, however, that physicians can use good practical common medical sense in determining whether or not treatment is efficacious and, if it is not, then cease the treatment.

By "hopeless" is meant that the prognosis for life (not meaningful life) is very poor. The fact that someone may not return to "sapient or cognitive life" may or may not fulfill the requirement, depending on other medical factors, but in and of itself it does not. As was said by the Supreme Court of West Germany:

Where human life exists, human dignity is present to it; it is not decisive that the bearer of this dignity himself be conscious of it and knows personally how to preserve it.[34]

Withdrawal of treatment and the subsequent death of the patient under these circumstances is not violative of any law.

Court intervention is only necessary where the decision is against treatment and where there does exist life-prolonging or life-saving treatment.

In the case of children, treatment should be offered the mentally incompetent on the same basis it is offered to the normal child.[35] Treatment may not be withheld merely because it is extraordinary when it is at the same time life-saving.[36] There is a scandal brewing in our country concerning the non-treatment of defective children or as Professor Ramsey says, "the benign neglect of defective infants." The medical standard for letting defective children die must be the same standard as is applied to normal children.

Notes

1. Cal. Health and Safety Code Secs. 7185-7195 (1977).

2. Arkansas, Idaho, Nevada, Texas, North Carolina, New Mexico, Oregon; Ark.State.Ann Sec. 82-3801-3804 (1977); N.C. Gen.Stat. Sec. 90-320-322 (1977); Idaho Code, Sec. 39-4501 to 4508 (1977); Nev.Rev.Stat. Sec. 449. 540-690 (1977); Tex. Health Code Ann. Act. 4590h (1977); An Act Relating to Medical Treatment of Terminally Ill Patients, 33rd. Leg. 1st Sess, Ch. 287 1977, New Mexico Laws; Or.Rev.Stat. Sec. 97.050 et seq.

3. As of December, 1979.

4. Texas has dropped the provision that two weeks must elapse after diagnosis of terminal treatment before a directive can take effect. The 5 year limitation has also been removed. North Carolina has changed the brain death section and clarified a section that deals with

incompetency. It now allows a notary public to witness such wills.

5. Society for the Right to Die, Legislative Manual, 1978.

6. Early history statement from the Society for the Right to Die, Dec. 1979.

7. Quoted from fund-raising letter of Sidney D. Rosoff, President, Society for the Right to Die, Dec. 1979 (emphasis in original).

8. Society for the Right to Die, "Program for the 1980s."

9. Letter of executive director of Concern for Dying, A-J Rock Levinson (Mrs. Henry W. Levinson), 10-3-78.

10. Concern for the Dying Newsletter, Vol. 5 No. 3, Summer 1979, pp. 1-4.

11. Private correspondence.

12. Horan, D. J., and Marcen, T., "Death with Dignity and the Living Will," 5 Notre Dame Journal of Legislation (1978); reprinted as pamphlet by Americans United for Life, 230 N. Michigan Avenue, Suite 515, Chicago, Illinois, 60601.

13. *Ibid.* AUL pamphlet at pp. 7, 8.

14. Kamisar, Yale, *Some Non-Religious Views Against Proposed Mercy-Killing Legislation,* 42 Minn. L. Rev. 969-1042 (1958); printed also in *Death, Dying and Euthanasia,* edited by Horan, D.J. and Mall, D., University Publications of America, Inc., Washington, D.C., 1977.

15. See my article for greater detail, op. cit. footnote 12.

16. Barry Keane, the original sponsor of California's Natural Death Act, has introduced a bill to veto the original act and replace it with another. Senate Bill 700 introduced March 21, 1979 (SB700) allows a person to direct his physician to withhold medical treatment and requires that the physician follow such a directive or be guilty of unprofessional conduct. In addition, while the directive is effective only with terminal patients, terminal illness is redefined to eliminate the limitation to "imminent death." This act is applicable even where death is likely to result within as long as six months. As a consequence we can see the safeguards of the original act being eroded and the slippery slope to euthanasia starting.

17. Because of its brevity we are here setting the Arkansas Act out in its entirety:

BE IT ENACTED BY THE GENERAL ASSEMBLY OF THE STATE OF ARKANSAS

SECTION 1. Every person shall have the right to die with dignity and to refuse and deny the use or application by any person of artificial, extraordinary, extreme or radical medical or surgical means or procedures calculated to prolong his life. Alternatively, every person shall have the right to request that such extraordinary means be utilized to prolong life to the extent possible.

SECTION 2. Any person, with the same formalities as are required by the laws of this State for the execution of a will, may execute a document exercising such right and refusing and denying the use or application by any person of artificial, extraordinary, extreme or radical medical or surgical means or procedures calculated to prolong his life. In the alternative, any person may request in writing that all means be utilized to prolong life.

SECTION 3. If any person is a minor or an adult who is physically mentally unable to execute or is otherwise incapacitated from executing either document, it may be executed in the same form on his behalf:

(a) By either parent of the minor;

(b) By his spouse;

(c) If his spouse is unwilling or unable to act, by his child aged eighteen or over;

(d) If he has more than one child aged eighteen or over, by a majority of such children;

(e) If he has no spouse or child aged eighteen or over, by either of his parents;

(f) If he has no parent living, by his nearest living relative; or

(g) If he is mentally incompetent, by his legally appointed guardian. Provided, that a form executed in compliance with this Section must contain a signed statement by two physicians that extraordinary means would have to be utilized to prolong life.

SECTION 4. Any person, hospital or other medical institution which acts or refrains from acting in reliance on and in compliance with such document shall be immune from liability otherwise arising out of such failure to use or apply artificial, extraordinary, extreme or radical medical or surgical means or procedures calculated to prolong such person's life.

SECTION 5. All laws and parts of laws in conflict with this Act are hereby repealed.

18. Byrne, Robert M., *Compulsory Life Saving Treatment for the Competent Adult*, 44 Fordham L.Rev. 1 (1975).

19. Grisez, Germain, *Suicide and Euthanasia* in *Death Dying and Euthanasia*, op.cit. footnote 14 at pp. 742-811.

20. Society for the Right to Die, Legislative Manual (1976) at p. 95.

21. See e.g. Sec. 9 of the California Act.

22. *In the Matter of Karen Quinlan, an Alleged Incompetent*, 70 N.J. 10, 355 A2d 647 (1976).

23. At one point the *Quinlan* court did refer to Karen's right not to endure the unendurable "only to vegetate a few measurable months." Slip Opinion p. 34; also published in *Death Dying and Euthanasia*, op.cit. footnote 14 where this statement is made at p. 509; see also the court's discussion of the hopeless and the dying at p. 515.

24. For my critique of the *Quinlan* case, see *Death Dying and Euthanasia*, op.cit. footnote 14 at pp. 525-534.

25. *Superintendent of Belcher Town State School v. Joseph Saikewicz, Mass.; 370 N.E.2d 417 (1977).*

26. *Ibid.* at p. 422.

27. McCormick, Richard A. and Hellegers, Andre, *The Specter of Joseph Saikewicz; Mental Incompetence and the Law*, America, April 1, 1978, pp. 257-260.

28. *In the Matter of Shirley Dinnerstein, Mass. App., 380 N.E.2d 134 (1978).*

29. *Saikewicz*, 370 N.E.2d at p. 431, see also p. 428.

30. Op.cit. footnote 28.

31. *Ibid.* at p. 139.

32. *Custody of a Minor*, Mass.; 379 N.E. 2d 1053 (1978).

33. *Maine Medical Center v. Houle*, No. 74-145 Superior Court, Cumberland, Maine, dec. 2-14-74. See also: *In the Matter of Kevin Sampson*, 317 N.Y.S. 2d 641 (N.Y. Supreme Court 1972); *In the Matter of Webberlist*, 360 N.Y.S. 2d 873 (N.Y. Supreme Court 1974).

34. Gorby et al, *West German Abortion Decision: A Contrast to Roe v. Wade*, 9 The John Marshall Journal of Practice and Procedure 551-684 (1976) at 559, 560.

35. Ramsey, Paul, *Ethics at the Edge of Life*, Yale University Press, 1978, pp. 189-228.

36. See cases cited at footnote 33; See also MacMillan, Elizabeth, *Birth-Defective Infants: A Standard for Nontreatment Decision*, 30 Stanford Law Review 599-633 (1978).

A Catholic Historical Perspective on Prolonging Life Decisions

Reverend Thomas J. O'Donnell, S.J.

The just-completed decade of the 70's witnessed an unprecedented interest in the ethical, moral, legal and medical aspects of terminal illness which has resulted not only in a swatch of entirely new litigation and legislation but also in a flood of both popular and professional journalism on the subject.

An historical review of the long and rich tradition of Catholic thought on the subject of man's responsibility of trying to prolong his life when it is threatened by some emergent fact such as accident or illness is appropriate because so many of the current writers seem either to have ignored or to have been unaware of this earlier vein of ethical thinking from which the very terms that they use were mined.

For example, the well-known situation ethicist, Joseph Fletcher, twenty years ago wrote what might be called a landmark article (because it has been and still is so often quoted) in a popular journal.[1] It is the kind of writing which could well convey the impression that the problem of prolonging life in terminal illness is as recent as the invention of the respirator. Fletcher observes, "We are, however, becoming somewhat less irrational than our forebearers on this subject," refers pejoratively to "the 'theological era' of the past," and (like many others) uses the term "extraordinary means" apparently without any awareness of the almost five centuries of Catholic theological reflection which forged it as a technical term in the context of terminal illness. Limiting his historical references to Thomas Sydenham (1624-1689) and Friedrich Nietzsche (1844-1900), the earliest source of Catholic teaching that Fletcher mentions is his own contemporary, Pope Pius XII. His article continues to be quoted in the literature, as for example in O. Ruth Russell's *Freedom to Die.*[2]

And although Dr. Russell would like to (but admittedly with some doubts) consider St. Thomas More as "the father of the euthanasia movement,"[3] she likewise thinks that "it was Pope Pius XII who modified the traditional doctrine of suffering and expressed approval of what is generally called passive or negative euthanasia."[4]

Historical Review

As a matter of fact (if one might pick a certainly significant if somewhat arbitrary place to begin) the famous Dominican theologican, Francisco Vitoria (d. 1546) early addressed the question of prolongation of life in terminal illness. It was de Vitoria who had innovated the use of the *Summa Theologica* of Thomas Aquinas (d. 1274) as the basic theology text instead of the "Sentences" of Peter Lombard (d. 1160) at the University of Salamanca.

Vitoria, extrapolating the germinal ideas of Thomas Aquinas on the rights and responsibilities of a man in regard to his own life, maintained, in effect, that both food and medicines were natural means of preserving one's life but that the obligation to use them was limited by their efficacy in the particular circumstances. Thus he taught that man had a basic obligation to use these means to prolong his life, but that it was an obligation that could be negatived in some extreme circumstances if they were without efficacy or even if, because of a personal revulsion on the part of the individual, they would be considered efficacious but extremely repugnant.[5]

The best-known theologians of the next 200 years did little more than project Vitoria's views into the very limited medical armamentarium of their times. It is true that when Vitoria was teaching at Salamanca there were medical schools in some European universities, but the curriculum was mainly a study of Galen, Avicenna and

Averroes. Pharmacology was still botany (plus such things as ground-up vipers) and in some universities a student had to swear that he would not become a surgeon nor operate *cum ferro et igne.* Surgery slowly passed from the hands of barbers into the hands of physicians. Near the middle of the sixteenth century Ambroise Pare started as a barber and finished as surgeon to Henry II, Francis II and Charles IX, and was surprised to discover, quite by accident, that battle wounds were better served by bandages than boiling oil.

Yet the theologians of these years did establish a firm and generally accepted set of principles regarding life and death and the medical practice of their time, principles which even today, as applied to modern medicine, remain essentially unchanged and widely accepted.

Among the most prominent of the theologians who wrote on these problems during the sixteenth, seventeenth and early eighteenth centuries were the two great Dominicans, Soto and Banez, who, after Vitoria, were so much responsible for the revival of scholasticism in sixteenth-century Spain. Dominic Soto (d. 1650) had studied under St. Thomas of Villanova and been professor at Alcala and Salamanca, and Charles V's theologian at Trent. Dominigo Banez (d. 1604) studied at Salamanca, where he later began his teaching career under Soto. He taught at Avila, where he became the spiritual director of St. Theresa and remained so for twenty years, until her death. He also taught at Alcala, at Valladolid, and eventually succeeded his former professor, Bartolome de Medina, as chief theologian at Salamanca.

Moreover, there were the four contemporary Jesuits addressing the same problems. Francisco Suarez (d. 1616) was a well-known professor and prolific writer and is said to have had as much influence on the Jesuit resurgence of scholasticism in Spain as Vitoria had among the Dominicans. And there was his Jesuit compatriot, Thomas Sanchez (d. 1610) who enjoyed what was perhaps the unique but not inappropriate reputation of being a saintly novice-master but a somewhat lax moralist (because of his views on mental reservation). The Flemish Jesuit, Leonard Lessius, who had studied under Suarez and subsequently taught at Louvain, was in frequent correspondence with St. Robert Bellarmine and greatly esteemed by St. Francis deSales. In addition to these three, there was the Austrian Jesuit, Paul Laymann (d. 1635), whose writings on the problems of terminal illness were so much respected by St. Alphonsus Liguori, and who taught at Munich and Dilligen.

Nor did the problems of prolongation of life escape the pen of that other distinguished Jesuit, John Cardinal deLugo – the child prodigy who could read at the age of three and made a public defense in logic at the age of fourteen. DeLugo taught at Medina del Campo, at Valladolid and at Rome. Alphonsus Liguori ranked him with Thomas Aquinas, and Pope Benedict IV called him "a light of the Church." He died in Rome in 1660. Also in Rome there was Antonio Dianna (d. 1663) who was consultant to the Holy See for the Kingdom of Sicily.

Such were the scholars from all of the famous universities of Europe whose teachings, a century later, the great founder of the Redemptorists, St. Alphonsus Liguori, was to study and sift and evaluate and summarize. It was by their hands that the principles were forged: that man's responsibility for the gift of life demands that he use ordinary means to preserve his life, but need not always use extraordinary or very difficult means, unless in some special circumstances such as, for example, if his life is extremely important to the common good.

It is quite understandable that Liguori retained the example of an extraordinary means that others had used before him: the amputation of a leg. At the time of his death (1789) any major surgery was clearly an extraordinary, desperate, harrowing, and frequently unsuccessful attempt to prolong life. It was not until well into the second half of the next century, following Lister's introduction of antiseptic technique and the beginnings of general anesthesia (ether by Long and chloroform by Morton and Simpson) that the survival rate after amputation got above 50%, more or less. The few other invasions of the body that had been surgically accomplished were likewise drastic and excruciatingly painful, such as the crude lithotomies that were done. It is interesting to note that around 1900 the well known Jesuit moral theologian at the Gregorian University, Gennaro Bucceroni, to exemplify extraordinary means of prolonging life, was still using "the amputation of a leg" but now adding "or the incision of the abdomen to remove a stone."

It is interesting to note, moreover, that among the authors from whose writings Liguori distilled his principle of ordinary-vs.-extraordinary means, with leg amputation as an obvious example of the latter, deLugo seems to have been the only one who had not been quite ready to accept the example as all that obvious. It seems to have been with either remarkable foresight or an uncommon allowance for medical progress that two centuries before general anesthesia deLugo had noted, with regard to the amputation, that one "should permit that cure when the doctors indicate it as necessary, and when it can be done without intense pain." But he contraindicates the amputation "if it would be accompanied by very intense pain, because no one is obliged to use extraordinary and very difficult means to preserve his life."[6]

And if it was only deLugo who seems to have had such prudent and long-range foresight, we can certainly say that, at least for the most part, the best known moral theologians of the latter half of the nineteenth century and the early decades of the twentieth were "au courant" of the medical and surgical advances of their times, and very much took them into account. While it is true, as I have pointed out elsewhere,[7] that some of the manualists of this period were still content to merely quote Liguori, others were monitoring the advances of surgery with the added safeguards of aseptic technique and anesthesia, and were prepared to re-evaluate procedures as ordinary or extraordinary accordingly.

To look, even sketchily, at the development of American theological reflection paralleling the medical and surgical advances associated with William Halsted (d. 1922), Harvey Cushing (d. 1939), the brothers Mayo (d. 1939) and their contemporaries is to sense an objective fascination on the part of the theologians with the new surgical techniques, clinical therapies and breaking pharmacological wonders. This was an "objective fascination" in the sense that their concern was a largely unsuccessful attempt to classify these new products and procedures as objectively (or, in themselves) ordinary or extraordinary means for prolonging life, by criteria such as: easily available vs. rare, unusual vs. common, natural vs. artificial, inexpensive vs. expensive, painless vs. painful, and such. These criteria were indeed helpful, but ultimately proved elusive and unsatisfactory because they were being applied too much to the medical advances in themselves rather than also sufficiently in relation to the condition of the particular patient. In all of this there was an untested supposition that the whole growing range of new techniques and therapies should be identifiable as either ordinary or extraordinary means of prolonging life, and be tagged as such.

A milestone and turning point in this "let's-be-specific" attitude can be identified in the theological literature current at the midpoint of the present century. The question under discussion was whether or not intravenous feeding should be considered an ordinary or an extraordinary means of prolonging life. The case proposed was of a terminally ill patient in considerable pain which could be alleviated only briefly due to drug toleration, but whose life could be prolonged for several weeks by intravenous feeding. Father Joseph Sullivan considered the case in his dissertion, "Catholic Teaching on the Morality of Euthanasia."[8] Father Joseph Donovan, C.M., presented his views in the *Homiletic and Pastoral Review* (August 1949) and Father Gerald Kelly, S.J., took up the case in *Theological Studies* (June 1950). All of these theologians considered intravenous feeding an ordinary means of prolonging life, but both Kelly and Sullivan allowed that in certain circumstances it could be discontinued; Kelly because "the mere prolonging of life in the given circumstances seems to be *relatively* useless" and Sullivan because "an artificial means of preserving life may be an ordinary or an extraordinary means *relative to* the physical condition of the patient" (emphasis added).

These considerations led to my own suggestion, six years later, that since the perpetually continued clinical prolongation of one's life is obviously not an *absolute* end and responsibility to be achieved at any cost (since we are all destined to die), it is therefore an end and responsibility to be achieved and fulfilled *relatively,* thus suggesting that the key to the problem lay in the answer to the question: "relatively to what?"

Seeing life as the fundamental God-given context in which man exercises all his potentialities, I proposed a calculus of proportion between the effort required to preserve that fundamental context and the potentialities that still remained.[9]

Comment

Thus it seems evident that in the richness and diversity of the modern medical armamentarium in which the experimental and unusual constantly cross over into the routine and accepted, one cannot, for the most part, speak of therapies and techniques as *simply* ordinary or extraordinary, but only *relatively* so, i.e.: relative to the total mental, moral and physical condition and prognosis of the patient. And this, after all, is basically what Francisco de Vitoria had been saying, in his own context, 400 years before: that the obligation to prolong life was limited by the efficacy of the means in the particular circumstances. To put it most briefly: therapy should tend to cure or at least to relieve. When it ceases to do either, it ceases to be therapy.

Because this concept of relatively ordinary or relatively extraordinary means of prolonging life ranges across a wide spectrum of personal assessment and decision, sometimes on behalf of others, subsequent reflection has suggested to me the necessity of identifying a category of care for the totally helpless terminal patient which might be called "minimal means" (such as customary hygenic and nutritional support) and which must always be used because, given the nature of the human composite, the neglect of such minimal care would be tantamount to an act of positive destruction.

For example: a newborn might be so extremely and definitively compromised (as might be the case with a severe encephalic with multiple other complications) as to be seen as having so little potential for meaningful life that any and all life-prolonging measures might be judged to be relatively extraordinary. In such a case it would not follow that abandonment would be acceptable. The customary hygenic and sustaining procedures such as normal feeding (if this would be possible), clearing air passages, supplying warmth, etc., would, I believe, be mandatory. There is a point at which neglect becomes destructive.

An awareness of this concept of minimal means which must always be used is not only important in itself, but in the present context of ethical reflection it is an important indicator and reminder that moral judgments based on the proportion involved in the concept of relatively ordinary and relatively extraordinary means are not reducible to a situation ethic. The morality of the use or omission of therapeutic measures is not determined solely by motive and circumstance. The obligation to use minimal means establishes that euthanasia is absolutely excluded as an intrinsically wrong moral object. Only with that made clear do motive and circumstances become the operational determinants of the morality of using or not using particular means to prolong life in the context of a particular terminal illness.

This review and comment on the 400-year history of Catholic reflection regarding human life as gift and responsibility should make it evident that when Pope Pius XII delivered his landmark address to the International Congress of Anesthesiologists (Nov. 24, 1957) he was not being doctrinally innovative but merely adding papal approbation to the long developed Catholic tradition that had preceded him and applying it to his contemporary medical context.

Notes

1. Joseph Fletcher, "The Patient's Right to Die," *Harper's Magazine,* October 1960, pp. 139-143.

2. O. Ruth Russell, *Freedom to Die* (New York: Human Sciences Press, rev. ed. 1977), p. 45.

3. *Ibid.,* p. 211.

4. *Ibid.,* p. 212.

5. I am indebted to Gary Atkinson, Ph.D., of the Pope John Center for the Aquinas-Vitoria point of departure for these observations.

6. *De Jure et Justitia,* disp. 10, n. 21 (Lyons 1670).

7. *Medicine and Christian Morality* (New York: Alba House, 1976), pp. 49-50.

8. Catholic University, 1949.

9. Thomas J. O'Donnell, S.J., *Morals in Medicine* (Westminster: The Newman Press, 1956).

Ethical Aspects of Decision and Consent in Terminal Illness

Reverend Thomas J. O'Donnell, S.J.

It may seem facetious and irrelevant to point out the obvious fact that death is much more definitive than a double-blind experiment. The point is that while, in recent years, perhaps almost equal amounts of ethical ink have been spent writing about the two topics of prolongation of life in terminal illness and human experimentation in clinical research, the question of informed consent has been exhaustively studied in relation to human experimentation but considerably neglected in regard to the prolongation of life in terminal illness.

While there are those who oppose euthanasia on the true, straightforward and uncomplicated moral grounds that the physician should not kill the patient, there are others who see a bit of merciful death-dealing as part of the role of the good physician but (they would say) only with the informed consent of the patient! To feel free to kill but scruple about consent may be admirable in some way, but suggests a rather bizarre priority of ethical values.

It is not my purpose here to treat the moral aspects of so-called positive and negative euthanasia (a new terminology that is unfortunate in that it implies a vastly lesser difference between killing and letting die than is verified in fact), but rather to reflect only on the place of consent in the decision to use or not to use extraordinary means to prolong life in an individual case.

Confronted with the medically doomed patient of negative prognosis, there are those who would claim that it is the prerogative of the physician to decide if and when these extraordinary and highly sophisticated means of prolonging life should be withdrawn. Others feel that this decision should be left to the next-of-kin. Actually, under normal circumstances and always basically, it is the prerogative of the patient to make these decisions.

The recognition of the individual's right to give free and informed consent to actions affecting his person (often called "the individual's right to self-determination") is basic to the Judeo-Christian tradition and the philosophy on which our way of life is founded. And the point of the earlier observation about death and double-blind experiments is that, if my consent is required for relatively harmless experimentation or clinical research on my person, it is evident that *a fortiori* my consent is required for withdrawing therapeutic measures (or abstaining from initiating them) and thus curtailing somewhat the prolonging of my life. Inalienable responsibilities, as well as inalienable rights, flow from the concept of "created equal."

The question of decision by next-of-kin or physician arises only when the patient is unable to make the decision. The inability on the part of the patient to make his own decision in his own case may be due to terminal coma, extreme weakness, or even such emotional instability that it is prudently judged this would render the decision-making a burden too heavy for the patient to bear. Under these circumstances if a decision is to be made (and it must be made, because in the very nature of the ongoing exigency, not to make a decision is, in itself, to decide one way or the other), it obviously must be made by someone other than the patient.

If the patient had previously delegated someone, as for example a relative or a physician, to make the decision in the event of these circumstances arising, then clearly the one delegated is acting as a qualified proxy and makes his own decision guided by his own judgment. But if, as is frequently the case, the decision is left to another simply by the default of the patient's ability to make it, then the decision should be an interpretative one — seeking what the patient would likely decide. (Note: Here we are dealing with adult patients. In the case of an infant, of course, the parents or those in their place have both the responsibility and the right to make the decisions in accord with the moral law.) But in the case of the interpretative decision, the decision must be made in accord with what is known of the patient's wishes in the context of the reasonable alternatives.

One must also be aware of the possibility that the physician subconsciously generates (or seems to generate) an unfortunate aura of iatrogenic proprietorship over the patient. This is usually idiomatic ("my patient") rather than actual ("I will decide what is good for you") and only overtones the physician's deeply personal interest in his patient. But where there are valid options, his medical ideal might conflict with what the family feels is more compassionate by letting the patient die in peace. It should only be noted that the "my patient" idiom does not include the prerogative of the physician to make all the decisions.

On the other hand, of course, there are some suppositions which favor the physician as a partner in the decision-making process, even beyond the intimate doctor-patient relationship of the family physician. It is the physician who is familiar with the reasonable medical alternatives, and who will be better able to judge both the cost of continued extraordinary care and the anticipated emotional strain on the family as the final illness is slowed down to what may be, for them, a tortured, drawn out, unproductive waiting while nature's merciful relief is being held off by sophisticated and useless technologies.

These then, are some of the parameters of decision and consent in the relationship of the terminally ill and the prolonging of life by extraordinary means, and here I have prescinded from the possible legal aspects of these questions and approached them only from a moral and ethical viewpoint. I have tried to outline the order of prerogatives of those who are called upon to make an interpretative decision of what the patient would want. In the last analysis it would seem that ideally the family, the physician, and perhaps some other intimate of the patient might best approach the decision together – with the final decision being the interpreted wishes of the patient, and not their own.

The "Living Will"

Reverend Thomas J. O'Donnell, S.J.

Currently statutory efforts with regard to the "living will" and "death with dignity" legislation merit special consideration because, while appearing to be highly idealistic and indeed almost a canonization of Catholic teaching on the use of ordinary and extraordinary means of prolonging life in terminal illness, they do in fact (and quite to the contrary) presage a dangerous and fairly subtle undermining of sound moral doctrine.

The "living will" is envisioned as a postulational (but eventually to-be-legalized) document whose purpose (eventually under the umbrella of "death with dignity" legislation) is supposedly to protect the right of the patient to refuse extraordinary means of prolonging life in terminal illness.

Euthanasia

The prototype of the living will, as conceived and distributed by the Euthanasia Educational Council (1972) is:

TO MY FAMILY, PHYSICIAN, MY CLERGYMAN, MY LAWYER: If the time comes when I can no longer take part in decisions for my own future, let this statement stand as a testament of my wishes: If there is no reasonable expectation of my recovery from physical or mental disability, I _____ request that I be allowed to die and not be kept alive by artificial means or heroic measures. Death is as much a reality as birth, growth, maturity and old age – it is the one certainty. I do not fear death as much as I fear the indignity of the deterioration, dependence and hopeless pain. I ask that drugs be mercifully administered to me for terminal suffering even if they hasten the moment of death.

This request is made after consideration. Although this document is not legally binding, you who care for me will, I hope, feel morally bound to follow its mandate. I recognize that it places a heavy burden of responsibility on you, and it is with the intention of sharing that responsibility and of mitigating any feelings of guilt that this statement is made. [There follows place for the signature and the date, and the signatures of two witnesses.]

A sufficient first alert should be recognized in the fact that the organized proponents of euthanasia in the United States have been largely responsible for initiating and pushing the living will. In 1975 the Euthanasia Educational Council reported that they had distributed three quarters of a million copies of their draft of the living will. That this is a strategy to pave the way toward legalized euthanasia is not just a Cassandra-cry from suspicious Catholics. In this regard it is interesting to note that O. Ruth Russell, Ph.D. (of Western Maryland College), one of the most articulate advocates of legalized euthanasia, in the recent revision of her book, *Freedom to Die*[1], complains that: "Some Catholics have been stepping up their opposition to the use of the living will," and quotes Father Joseph Hogan, C.M., of St. John's University, New York, as accusing the Euthanasia Council of using the living will as a form of propaganda to form the public mind according to its point of view (pp. 382-3).

This somewhat pejorative-sounding report of Catholic suspicions becomes even more interesting when we note that, earlier in her same book, Dr. Russell observes that in the 1960's the Euthanasia Society of America did not press for legislation because "further efforts toward legalization would be futile until a more favorable climate of opinion has been created" and so "the board adopted a policy of limiting its efforts to education rather than legislation" (p. 180). Dr. Russell points out that the next step of the Euthanasia Society was to set up the Euthanasia Educational Fund (1967), the name of which was changed as above, with the mass distribution of the living will. Dr. Russell further observes: "The publicity given to the Living Will has helped promote discussion of euthanasia: it has also had the positive effect of making doctors more aware of the current support for voluntary euthanasia" (p. 182).

Further evidence of this subtle strategy was noted by Bishop Ernest Unterkoefler of Charleston in his public statement opposing this type of legislation in South Carolina (Jan. 13, 1977):

> ... Dr. Florence Clotheir, a member of the board of directors of the Euthanasia Educational Council, has stated that once the principle of passive euthanasia is established by the living will legislation it will be necessary for society "to confront the greater dilemmas inherent in active euthanasia for the hopelessly malformed and handicapped infants doomed to a bestial subhuman existence in our state institutions. Active euthanasia may also have its place for patients suffering from incurable, intractable pain, but for the present there are dilemmas enough in regard to passive euthanasia."[2]

Patient Rights

Not only is living-will and death-with-dignity legislation seen by some of its most ardent proponents as a necessary first step toward legalized euthanasia, but there is indeed another yet more subtle danger inherent in it. While it is being presented as legislation designed to protect the rights of the patient, its effect is rather to confer certain legal immunities on the physician. Moreover these immunities, at least possibly by implication, tend to expand the rights of the physician beyond their actual scope and to the possible detriment of the rights of the patient, or at least the patient's ready exercise of those rights.

The right of the patient (or the family, acting for the incompetent patient) to refuse extraordinary means of prolonging life which are useless and perhaps even damaging to the patient's total good, is a right which is already clear from the natural law and is adequately recognized and protected in civil law by the canons of informed consent for any kind of treatment. And even though death-with-dignity and living-will legislation is proposed merely as a statutory articulation of that right in the particular circumstances of terminal illness, it might well come to be understood as a legal conferral of the right itself; which would thus imply the power of the state to also withhold that right.

This is a danger which is indeed neither fictitious nor negligible. It may even be part of the reason why so many of those who promote positive euthanasia are so supportive of this type of legislation. It is certainly a subtle step in the direction of their ultimate design. It should be clear that the recognition of legislation as necessary or appropriate to restrain a physician from treating a patient under specific circumstances carries a deceptive and dangerous implication that is far removed from the ordinary canons of consent.

In an excellent article published in 1977, Richard McCormick, S.J., and Andre Hellegers, M.D., pointed out that this kind of legislation subtly seems to shift the *locus* of the right to make decisions regarding treatment (at least in terminal illness) away from the patient (or family) and into the hands of the physician, unless opposed by legal instrument.[3]

Not only do the present canons of informed consent protect the patient's right to refuse treatment but, as Bishop Walter F. Sullivan of Richmond pointed out some years ago in his pastoral letter, " 'Death with Dignity' Ministry, not Legislation," the living will concept actually tends to violate these canons. Bishop Sullivan wrote:

> The concept of the "living will" also raises a serious issue of whether a person is capable of real "informed consent" to such a document. The question is, "How do I determine far in advance of a terminal illness my feelings about death at the time of death?" It is very hard to imagine that we really know what we think about death when we are healthy and perhaps in the prime of our lives. It is questionable, therefore, whether we can actually sign a document which will validly express our future feelings and concerns about death. Valid "informed consent" requires that an individual have necessary information about the intended medical treatment – details of the procedures, benefits, alternative procedures, and so on – before direction or consent is given to the physician. Obviously this is not possible with a "living will" since the exact nature of the possible terminal conditions is unknown at the time consent is given.

Legal Language

There is also the problem, of course, inherent in freezing what are necessarily imprecise moral and medical technical terms into fixed and only apparently precise legal language. Such terms as "reasonable expectation of recovery," "physical or mental disability," "artificial means," "extraordinary measures," etc., are much too fluid to be fixed into legal language. Terminal illness often presents delicate human and moral questions and situations which can be clarified only in the patient-physician-family relationship and which (as Bishop Sullivan also pointed out) cannot be reduced to legal and juridical concepts without provoking litigations, inadequate definitions, ambiguous notions, and further equally unsuccessful legislation, as has been recently demonstrated in the California legislature. As Professor Robert Audi of the University of Nebraska at Lincoln recently pointed out: "But having affirmed all these rights, I would emphasize that it is best if doctors and their patients try to structure their relationships so that the *assertion* of rights on either side is unnecessary."[4]

Notes

1. New York: Human Sciences Press, 1977.

2. Florence Clothier, *Euthanasia: The Physician's Dilemma* (New York: Euthanasia Educational Council, 1972), pp. 2f. *Origins* 7, 34 (Feb. 9, 1978): 543-44.

3. "Legislation and the Living Will," *America,* March 12, 1977, pp. 210-213.

4. *Contemporary Issues in Biomedical Ethics,* edited by J. Davis, B. Hoffmaster and S. Shorten (Clifton: The Humana Press, 1978), p. 62.

Theological and Pastoral Dimensions of Prolonging Life Decisions

Reverend Donald G. McCarthy, Ph.D.

In this final essay on prolonging life issues the focus will be on contemporary efforts to describe which means of prolonging life are to be considered morally obligatory in the Catholic tradition of stewardship of human life. Several related questions will be addressed very briefly at the end of this chapter.

The Ethical Distinction of Ordinary and Extraordinary Means

The classical definition in Catholic moral theology for an ethically extraordinary means of prolonging life is "all medicines, treatments, and operations, which cannot be obtained or used without excessive expense, pain, or other inconvenience for the patient or for others, or which, if used, would not offer a reasonable hope of benefit to the patient."

There is some effort in the present state of renewal and re-evaluation of Catholic moral theology to move beyond the term "extraordinary" means of prolonging life. But no suitable substitute term has emerged thus far. In the previous discussion earlier in this book I proposed the term "Justifiable Use of Conservative Therapy Only" (JUCTO) for situations where extraordinary means of prolonging life are omitted. Regardless of terminology, the decisive factor determining if a medical procedure actually is ethically extraordinary will hinge on the "benefit" it offers the patient or the "burden" it imposes.

If we pick out that specific question of "benefit," we can ask how we determine when there is an insufficient benefit to obligate us morally to use some life-prolonging procedure? I have already suggested two cases when benefit becomes minimal: when death is imminent or when a person is in the grips of a coma known with medical certainty to be irreversible. There may still be special circumstances enhancing this minimal benefit: for example, if a person has not made his or her peace with God this would be a pastoral reason to prolong life as long as possible. But at least as a general statement, when death is imminent we can see minimal benefit in prolonging life, particularly when one is suffering at the moment of death. Irreversible coma likewise comes to be accepted as a version of minimal benefit.

Let us now consider several actual cases where some medical procedure may be considered ethically extraordinary and could be omitted within the tradition of respecting life. The first is from literature in England, used in two different articles, and in both of them cited as a reason why England should legalize mercy killing to avoid this kind of tragic case.

Dr. C is dying of cancer and everything possible has been done for him. Then he has a cardiac arrest, but has cardiopulmonary resuscitation (CPR) five times, and lingers several more weeks with convulsions because of the anoxia, lack of oxygen to the brain, during the arrests which brought on brain damage.

My question is, could we not practice "Justifiable Use of Conservative Therapy Only" and allow this man to die, rather than resuscitate him five times so that he can die a total of six times? He was a physician and it was his own colleagues who were resuscitating him even though he was asking to be allowed to die. This presents a horrible example, but I don't think we should presume that these kinds of tragic situations are happening every day. That would create an unwarranted panic mentality. But we do have a sample of the problem arising from an exaggerated form of medical scrupulosity using a treatment not beneficial to the patient. I suspect Dr. Collins would not consider this good medicine, to resuscitate this man who is hopelessly dying of cancer and in the last stages of his terminal illness.

A second case is the Karen Quinlan case and it raises the issue of JUCTO as well as the issue of consent. She was not a minor, she was over 21, and that led to some of the court considerations on the guardianship question. The court is concerned about crime: the omission of ethically ordinary care of someone entrusted to our care can be considered homicide by omission, a crime. Would the turning off of the respirator, if she had died shortly afterward, have been a criminal action? One doctor in my home town assured me, in the way that only Zeus speaks on Mt. Olympus, that turning off a respirator is exactly the same as cutting one's throat. I don't believe that is true, hence this offers a case to be considered.

The third case is a true one from a hospital where the nursing supervisor was aware of the case and described it to me. The patient was a 90-year-old woman, completely senile, with asthma, bronchitis, pneumonia and congestive heart failure, who had received antibiotics and a tracheotomy, and was on a respirator. She then had a cardiac arrest and was resuscitated contrary to the family's wishes by a young physician. The young physician, of course, can be lauded for his respect for life but we may wonder if that was a morally good decision, especially since he made it contrary to those who spoke for the patient.

Could this woman not have been allowed to die? Notice that there is a constellation of factors here. We would not propose a blanket policy of no resuscitation for anyone 90 years of age. That obviously does not consider the individual benefit to the patient. Some years ago a hospital in England put through a policy that they would not resuscitate anyone over 65 years of age. That might help the Social Security budget but it doesn't seem to be a humane practice of medicine.

Having mentioned those kinds of cases, we might sketch some cases where the omission of medical procedures would be morally wrong because it is the omission of ordinary means of prolonging life. These would be examples of omissions which would fit under that unacceptable term "passive euthanasia" which, in a respect-life tradition, would be objectional omissions.

One example is not strictly medical. Consider a couple who is caring for an aged mother of the husband. She is a burden and on a given Saturday night after a particularly irritating day she has gone to the bathroom for her bath. They hear a thud, she has slipped in the tub, hit her head and is sliding gently beneath the surface of the water. The couple open the door and, viewing her, look at each other in relief because their problems are solved. Not to extract her from the water would be a form of omission. There would be no action whatsoever. But it would very likely be a homicidal situation because of the neglect of a very basic responsibility to the mother-in-law. We would consider this criminal negligence or omission.

An analogy to this in medicine might be found in the case of a woman who is in reasonably good health, perhaps in her forties. She is extremely depressed and bereaved by the sudden death of her husband. She decides not to take her insulin to control her diabetes. If she is in generally good health and in mid-life, we would be inclined to say that the insulin is part of her responsibility to care for the gift of her life. Psychologically, she may not be fully aware of the decision she is making. She may be emotionally disturbed, but looking at her action objectively in terms of care of life, I would say that hers would be a morally objectionable omission; the insulin would be considered ordinary care. Her omission, while not an act of commission, would be equivalent to the suicidal act of self-destruction. This leads to the discussion of which omissions are suicidal and which are not? If Karen Quinlan had been able to ask for removal of the respirator (despite her coma) we may not have considered that suicidal.

Another example might be a woman in mid-life with breast cancer who had a 98% chance of recovery through a mastectomy but, because of vanity or fear, does not make the choice of surgery. That could be considered omitting an ordinary means of prolonging life, given various factors.

The really critical problem, then, in contemporary discussion is this: what will be the criteria for ordinary and extraordinary means of prolonging life? How shall we set up the measurement of benefit? The real danger which most of us see, I believe, is to drift into this mentality: IF WE CANNOT RETURN THIS PATIENT TO "NORMAL" LIFE, OUR MEDICAL PROCEDURES ARE EX-TRAORDINARY. I believe that is a trap. It leads into a definite form of elitism where everyone who is subnormal is unwelcome in terms of medical treatment.

If we talk about this key issue of benefit from medical treatment, we might envision four kinds of situations where a person may be very possibly on a plateau in terms of future prognosis: neither improvement not deterioration expected.

These four kinds of situations would come from: a low I.Q., senility, paralysis, helplessness. Considering each one in terms of possible future developments we have the following expectations:

1. The low I.Q. will probably neither improve nor deteriorate but remain the same;

2. Senility probably won't improve but it might deteriorate or remain the same;

3. Paralysis might improve, remain the same, or deteriorate;

4. Various kinds of medical helplessness might also improve, remain the same, or deteriorate.

Here is the point of this outline. If we say that those procedures which help to improve will be likely ethically *ordinary* and that if, despite our treatment, a person is going to deteriorate, so that the treatment might be lacking in sufficient benefit and ethically *extraordinary,* what shall we say about our treatment when the person will simply remain on the same plateau? In our pragmatic society there is a great tendency to say that if a person is going to remain the same, and that is subnormal, he need not be treated. We see that in terms of how some surgeons, for example, are inclined not to perform surgery on the mentally retarded. I do not believe our Christian tradition of a morally equal dignity of all persons supports a discriminatory omission of medical treatment simply on the basis that a person's "quality of life" remains on a subnormal plateau. This needs careful discussion.

Related Questions

Categories of care are now being used in some hospitals distinguishing four levels ranging from full and total use of all available procedures to omission of everything but minimal care and comfort. Such classifications are not in themselves objectionable but the ethical challenge is to make them with maximum accuracy according to moral norms and with proper consent of the patient or patient's representative.

The "Christian Affirmation of Life" was designed and published by the Catholic Health Association to help people think about prolonging-life issues. It is a document to record in Christian language one's disposition to omit ethically extraordinary means of prolonging life. It does not make any legally definitive judgment and is not intended to be made a legal document by statute law. It is an educational and contemplative, meditative kind of document which can be of great help in pastoral ministry.

With regard to documents intended to be legal instruments I would note, first of all, that we have a human right to forego unreasonable treatment but not to manipulate death. Some problems arise when the Living Will is made legally binding and they have been reviewed by Mr. Dennis Horan and Father Thomas O'Donnell (pp. 152-159 and 173-177).

A further problem arises because many of the sponsors of Living Will legislation are also in the camp of legalizing active euthanasia eventually, or they do not see a moral difference between active euthanasia and omissions of life-prolonging measures, even those carefully described here as ethically extraordinary. It is time to conclude and I do so, recalling a basic Christian theme, responsible and reverential stewardship of human life.

Index

Gaudium et Spes, 5
Genesis, 3
Gide, Andre, *quoted,* 103-104
Genetic diagnosis, 12
    and abortion, 91-92
Genetic surgery, 47
Griffin, Dr. John, xii

HEW, 46, 105
Health care, xiv, xv
Hillebrand, Rev. Wilhelm, 38
Hormones:
    FSH, 30
    LH, 30
Hoyt, Robert, *quoted,* 69
Hominization, delayed, 85
Hospice movement, 152
Houle case, 158
Humanae Vitae, 20, 23, 41, 57, 70
Humanism, secular:
    in America, 89-90, 96n
Hybrids, 11

IUD, *see* Intrauterine device
Implantation (nidation), 35-36, 49
In vitro fertilization, 10, 11, 43-46, 64, 67-68
Informed consent, 170-172, 176
Intrauterine device, 9-10, 48-50
    copper-clad, 49
    polyethylene, 48-49
    progesterone, 49-50
Irreversibility and death, 119, 124, 127-128

John XXIII, Pope, *quoted,* 5, 106-107
John Paul II, Pope, 57, 70, 90
    Quoted, ix, 5, 6, 19, 56, 60, 73
Judiciary, *see* Courts
JUCTO (Justifiable Use of Conservative Therapy Only), 142, 179-180

Kamisar, Yale, 153
Kass, Leon, 133